LEAN
HEALTHCARE

How to trim fat and waste from your organization
while improving access, quality, and service

SCOTT LISBIN

TABLE OF CONTENTS

Chapter 1   Introduction and Overview   1

Chapter 2   How to Identify Waste   17

Chapter 3   How to Identify the Cause(s) of Waste   51

Chapter 4   How to Eliminate the Cause(s) of Waste   71

Chapter 5   How to Prevent Waste   221

Chapter 6   Leading Change   231

                Appendix   253

                Index   285

CHAPTER 1

Introduction and Overview

1.1   Do More With Less!

Do more with less! Sound familiar?

If you work as a manager for just about any healthcare organization, you have probably already been asked *(or soon will be)* to do "more with less" and "do it better".

Most healthcare organizations today find themselves fighting to attract and retain customers. These customers are more and more demanding and want to receive the highest quality care and service at the lowest possible price.

Most organizations have responded to these customer demands by putting increased pressure on their managers to both reduce costs and improve quality! If you are like most managers, you have probably thought how can I do "more with less" and still "do it better"?

The answer is you have to get "**LEAN**" and trim the fat and waste from your department or organization operations.

Why?

Because it is estimated that approximately $1 out of every $3 spent in the delivery of healthcare represents "**MUDA**" or "waste". [1]

1. Altarum, Healthcare Value Hub, https://www.healthcarevaluehub.org/advocate-resources/healthcare-waste.

LEAN HEALTHCARE

To increase access, quality, and service while reducing cost in your organization you will need to understand:

1. What *"Muda"* or "waste" is

2. How you can identify "waste"

3. How "waste" affects the costs and quality of healthcare

4. How you can determine the cause(s) of observed "waste"

5. What actions you can take to reduce or eliminate "waste" to reduce costs or improve quality or service

6. What actions you can take to prevent "waste"

7. How you can sustain the changes and improvements you make

If you follow the steps outlined in the following chapters you **will** have the knowledge and tools needed to get "**LEAN**" and "do more with less" and "do it better".

See appendix I for a listing of the six domains of healthcare quality.

1.2 Waste Not Want Not

It has been said that the worst type of "waste" is the "waste" which goes unseen.

Therefore, in order to reduce costs and improve quality and service it is important to understand what "waste" is and how to identify it.

"Waste" is referred to in Lean as *"MUDA"*, which is Japanese for wasteful or "no value" activities.

There are eight (8) types of *"MUDA"* which add to cost or reduce access, quality, or service.

These eight (8) types of *"MUDA"* include:

1. DEFECTS

Defects are errors or mistakes that require additional time, resources, or money to fix.

Defects include anything that has not been done correctly the first time and, in healthcare, include errors such as:

- Misdiagnosis

- Surgical errors (i.e., wrong side, site, procedure, or patient)

- Hospital acquired conditions (i.e., MRSA)

- Adverse outcomes or medication errors

- Falls or pressure ulcers

- Incorrect IDC codes

Healthcare typically measures errors as the number of defects per 100 or 1000 encounters (due to their high frequency) vs. industry which typically measures defects per 1,000,000 (due to their low frequency).

No matter the industry, the goal for any organization according Philip Crosby in his book *"Quality is Free"* should be "**zero**" defects.

2. WAITING

Waiting is any idle time produced when two interdependent processes are not completely synchronized.

Patients, staff, and clinicians are frequently required to "wait" because the next step in the process is not ready for them or required supplies, equipment, or resources are unavailable.

Waiting is one of the biggest sources of frustration for both patients, staff, and physicians and include:

- Patients waiting for an appointment to see a doctor

- Delays in fulfilling doctor's orders on a nursing unit

- Physicians and patients waiting for test results

- Patients waiting for an available bed following admission

- Patients waiting to be discharged once medically Cleared

Waiting is so prevalent in healthcare that Jay Arthur in his book

"A Faster Hospital in Five Days" contends that "**most**" (up to 95 percent) of a patient's time when receiving care or treatment is spent "**idle**" just waiting for something to happen.

3. OVERPRODUCTION

Overproduction is making or doing something too soon, making or doing too much of something, or making or doing something faster than needed.

Examples of overproduction in healthcare include:

- Scheduling of return clinic visits for all patients seen

- Performing mammograms on all adult female patients

- Changing unsoiled bed sheets daily on occupied patient beds

- Ordering inappropriate or unnecessary tests or procedures

- Routinely prescribing or overusing antibiotics

It is estimated that $1 out of every $10 dollars spent in the delivery of healthcare is "wasted" on unnecessary care or services".[2]

4. OVERPROCESSING

Overprocessing is putting more into a product or service than is valued by the customer.

In healthcare, overprocessing is often interpreted to mean making care or services more complex or expensive than necessary and is

2. Altarum, Healthcare Value Hub, https://www.healthcarevaluehub.org/advocate-resources/healthcare-waste.

often referred to as "**overtreatment**".

Unlike in other industries where there is usually only one customer, in healthcare there may be several customers; all with different concerns, interests, and priorities.

The customer in healthcare may be the patient, who often lacks the medical knowledge necessary to determine the "value" or "necessity" of the care or services provided, the healthcare provider, a third-party payor such as an insurance carrier or employer, or a governmental agency (i.e., Medicare or Medi-Cal).

Some of the most common examples of overprocessing or "**overtreatment**" in healthcare include:

- Keeping patients in the hospital longer than needed

- Ordering complex diagnostic imagery (i.e., MRI) when a simpler method would be sufficient (i.e., X-ray)

- Performing a surgical procedure in lieu of an equally effective and more conservative medical treatment

- Receiving treatment from a specialist when the treatment could have been provided by the patient's primary care physician

- Providing end of life patients with aggressive end of life care rather than hospice or palliative care

The amount of dollars being "wasted" on overprocessing or overtreatment of patients according to Donald Berwick, MD, in his article "Eliminating Waste in US Health Care" is estimated to total $1 out of every $20 dollars.[3]

3. Berwick et al. (2012). Eliminating Waste in US Health Care. *JAMA* 2012;307(14):1513-1516, https://jamanetwork.com/journals/jama/article-abstract/1148376

5. **MOTION**

Motion is defined as any excess movement, whether by employees or machines, that doesn't add value to the product, service, or process.

Wasted motion occurs very frequently in the delivery of healthcare; with staff and physicians "wasting" a lot of time searching for equipment, supplies, or information required for care of the patient.

Poorly laid out facilities, inefficient procedures, and outdated technologies also contribute to "wasted" movement and motion; resulting in additional lost staff and physician time and productivity.

Examples of "wasted" motion in healthcare include:

- Searching for critical labs or notes in a patient's medical record

- Searching for missing surgical instruments, equipment, or supplies

- Manually entering lengthy passwords rather than using RFID technology for computer security access authentication

- Manually entering orders rather than using standardized order sets or smart phrases

- Performing manual inventory count rather than using scanning technology

According to various studies, as much as 20% of a nurse's day is spent searching for equipment, supplies, or other items or information needed to take care of their patients.[4]

4. Pronovost et al. (2019). Improving Hospital Productivity as a Means to Reducing Costs. *Health Affairs* March 26, 2019, https://www.healthaffairs.org/do/10.1377/hblog20190321.822588/full/

6. **TRANSPORTATION**

Transportation is the movement of things from one location to another.

Transportation of many things is required in the delivery of healthcare.

Patients, supplies, medications, and equipment are frequently moved throughout clinics and hospitals in order to provide patients with the care they require.

Some common examples of transportation in healthcare include:

- Moving a patient from the ICU to a step-down unit

- Moving supplies from the central storeroom to the nursing unit where it is needed for patient care

- Moving a C-Arm from one OR suite to another

- Taking blood and urine specimens to the lab for processing

While not adding value to either the patient care experience or clinical outcomes, transportation is often an "**essential**" non-value activity which may not be able to be eliminated because of the need for access to costly and specialized equipment (i.e., MRI, CT, etc.) and/or services (i.e., blood bank, ORs, etc.).

7. **INVENTORY**

Inventory consists of the materials, supplies, and products being held in storage or being used in the manufacture of a product or delivery of a service.

According to one study of hospital costs, materials and supplies account for about 15% of all hospital costs.[5]

Examples of healthcare inventory include:

- Drugs being stored in the pharmacy or on the nursing units for patient care

- Surgical instruments, custom packs, and instrument trays being stored in Central Processing or the Operating Room for use during surgery

- Saline solution, syringes, and needles being stored in Central Distribution for later distribution to the nursing units for patient care

According to some studies, up to 30% of a hospital's inventory of supplies expire, become obsolete, or end up being wasted.[6]

In healthcare, unlike in other industries, inventory is not just limited to materials and supplies.

Healthcare organizations also have inventories of appointments, hospital beds, and OR block time that need to be effectively managed.

Effective management of these inventories is as important as

5. Abdulsalam et al. (2017). Hospital supply expenses: An important ingredient in health services research. *Medical Care Research and Review*, 1-13, published on line, July 24, 2017
https://hmpi.org/2017/09/09/how-much-do-u-s-hospitals-spend-on-medical-supplies/

6. Inventory: A Hidden Asset in Healthcare. Suture Express. July 28, 2017
https://blog.sutureexpress.com/inventory-hidden-asset-healthcare

effective management of supply inventories; as poor management of these inventories can be even more costly in terms of lost revenue, delayed access to required treatment, and increased patient dissatisfaction.[7]

8. HUMAN TALENT

Waste of human talent is the inappropriate utilization or underutilization of staff and/or physician time, skills, knowledge, or ideas.

Unlike many industries, healthcare is heavily reliant on human talent for the delivery of care and services; with staff and physicians typically accounting for 60% or more of a hospital's or clinic's total expenses.

Despite its operational importance and cost, human talent frequently ends up being "wasted" through either inefficient, ineffective, or inappropriate utilization.

Some common examples of human talent "waste" include:

- A physician providing care that could have been provided by a nurse practitioner or physician assistant

- A physician who sees only 70% of the total number of patients that should be seen in a half day

- A financial analyst preparing a report that nobody uses

- An idea for improvement shared by an employee that is ignored or not even considered

7. Patient Throughput: A Critical Strategy for Success, The Chartis Group, White Paper Fall 2007
http://www.chartis.com/resources/files/whitepapers/pre-2013/chartis_group_patient-throughput-critical-strategy-for-success.pdf

- An employee that is idle or not doing anything productive

Various studies estimate the loss from hospital inefficiencies and its associated waste of human talent at between 11% and 25% of total hospital costs.[8]

Given how prevalent waste is throughout the healthcare system, is there "waste" or "*MUDA*" in your department or organization?

8. Mutter et al. (2008). Measuring Hospital Inefficiency: The Effects of Controlling for Quality and Patient Burden of Illness. *Health Services Research*, 2008, Dec, 43(6): 1992 -2013
https://www.ncbi.nlm.nih.gov/pmc/articles/PMC2614001/

1.3   A Model Approach

One of the best ways to initially determine if there are *any* opportunities for improvement in your department or organization is to do an assessment.

An assessment is usually the first step in the performance improvement process used by most organizations.

The **Plan, Do, Study/Check, Act** (PDSA or PDCA) model is one of the most common performance improvement models used in both manufacturing and healthcare.

Another model which clinicians can often more readily relate to is the **Assess, Diagnose, Treat, and Prevent** model shown below since it parallels the way many clinicians approach their daily work.

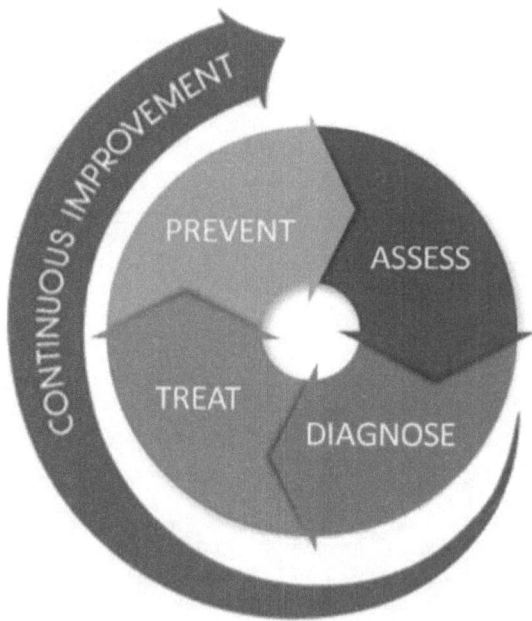

Note: "Examine" can be used in place of "Assess".

LEAN HEALTHCARE

Using this model, the first step in the process improvement model is to perform an examination or assessment.

There are a number of different ways to assess whether or not there are *any* opportunities for reduction or elimination of "*MUDA*" or "waste" in *your* department or organization.

Some of the most common approaches for doing this assessment include:

- Walking the *gemba*

- Preparing a process map

- Preparing a value stream map

- Benchmarking

- Using computer simulation

- Utilizing customer feedback

Note: Six Sigma uses the Define, Measure, Assess, Improve, Control model.
See appendix II for more information on this model and the differences between Six Sigma and LEAN.

ASSESS

Making Waste Visible

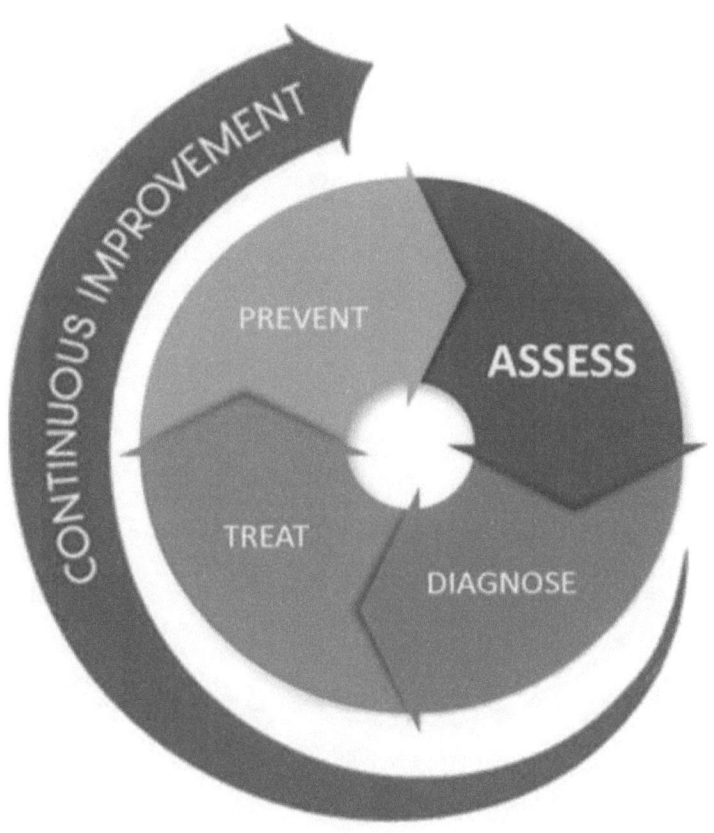

CHAPTER 2
How to Identify Waste

2.1   Make Waste Visible

Before "waste" or *"MUDA"* can be reduced or eliminated in your department or organization, you must first be able to "see" it.

Sometimes the presence of "waste" is obvious and easy to "see" such as when employees are sitting idle or having to walk long distances to get supplies or equipment.

At other times "waste" can be more difficult to "see" such as when physician orders are delayed in being written or fulfilled or when clinician treatment practices vary.

So how can the "waste" in your department or organization be made visible?

Some of the most common approaches utilized to make "waste" or *"MUDA"* more visible include:

- Walking the *"gemba"*

- Preparing a process map

- Preparing a value stream map

- Benchmarking

- Using computer simulation

- Utilizing customer feedback

- Work sampling

These approaches vary significantly in their ease of use and application; from some needing little training to successfully apply (i.e., *gemba* walk), to other methods that require extensive training (i.e., computer simulation).

Whether "walking the *gemba*" or "preparing a process map", use of these different techniques will help make "waste" more visible in order to identify opportunities for reduction or elimination of "*MUDA*".

And that means being able to do more with less and do it better!

2.2   Walk the *Gemba*

"*Gemba*" is the Japanese word for "actual place".

Walking the "*gemba*" or going to the location where the work is actually performed, is one of the best ways to do an assessment and identify potential "waste".

When "walking the *gemba*" it is important to observe the work being performed and look for some of the "**telltale signs**" that frequently signal problems with "*MUDA*" or "waste" in an organization.

Some of the most common "telltale signs" of "waste" include:

- Piles of work that are backlogged or not being worked on

- Patients that are waiting for service or care

- Staff or clinicians that are sitting idle or unable to do their work because they are waiting for patients or results

- Staff or clinicians that are looking for information, supplies, or other items that they need to do their jobs

- Problems or bottlenecks in workflow

- Staff or clinicians that have to redo work that's already been done because it wasn't done properly the first time

- Staff or clinicians not following the prescribed policies or procedures

- Frequent complaints from customers or patients

- Staff or clinicians looking rushed or harried

- Troughs and/or peaks in demand.

Seeing some, if not all, of these telltale signs when "walking the *gemba*" is to be expected...as there are opportunities to eliminate or reduce "waste" in almost every department or organization.

If the presence of "waste", however, isn't uncovered by "walking the *gemba*", it doesn't mean that everything is running great and there isn't any "waste".

It just means that a different tool may be needed to help make the presence of any "waste" visible.

2.3 Process Mapping

People absorb information in different ways.

Some people absorb information visually, others absorb information aurally, and still others absorb information kinesthetically (i.e., by doing).

Most people, however, are visual and able to better absorb, retain, and analyze information by seeing it rather than by hearing it or even experiencing it *(note: studies indicate 65% of people are visual learners)*.[9]

Therefore, process maps can be powerful tools to help identify opportunities for reduction of "*MUDA*" or "waste".

A process map or flowchart is a visual representation of the sequence of steps and decisions needed to perform a task or process (see example below).

A BASIC FLOWCHART

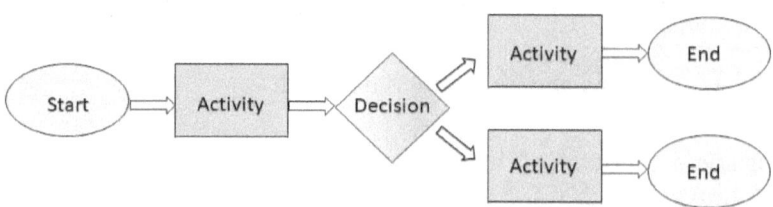

Flowcharting a task or process helps make any redundant, inefficient, or unnecessary steps which would be considered "waste" stand out and more "visible".

Different symbols or "blocks" are typically used to flowchart a task or process.

The most commonly used symbols include the six blocks shown on the following page.

9. St. Louis, M. (2017). How to spot visual, auditory, and kinesthetic-learning executives. *INC*, Aug 1,2017
https://www.inc.com/molly-reynolds/how-to-spot-visual-auditory-and-kinesthetic-learni.html

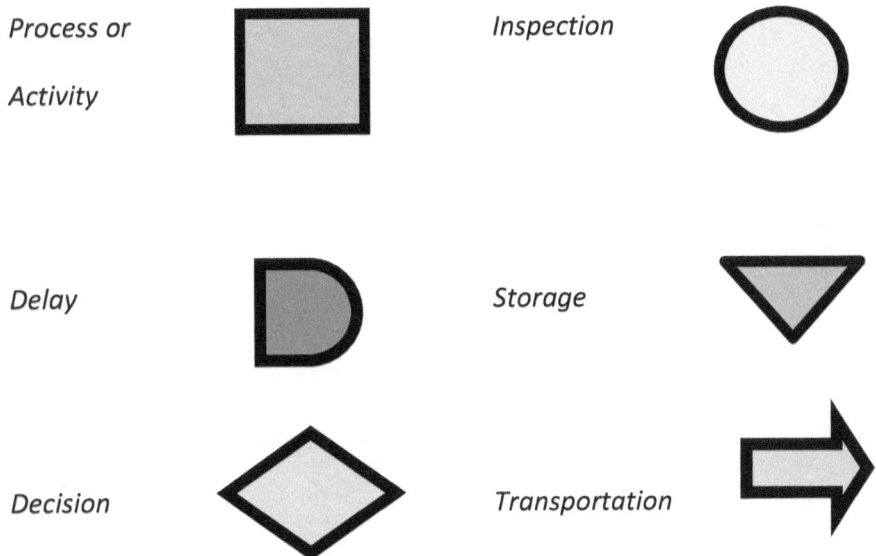

Process or Activity	[square]	Inspection	[circle]
Delay	[D shape]	Storage	[inverted triangle]
Decision	[diamond]	Transportation	[arrow]

These symbols, along with those in appendix III if needed, can be used to construct a flowchart by following the five simple (5) steps identified below:

1. Determine the start and end point for each task

2. Determine what type of flowchart to construct (see below for most common types of flowcharts)

3. Observe the task being performed

4. Document the actual steps performed for each task

5. Create a flowchart using the appropriate symbols for each step

Four types of flowcharts are typically used in healthcare to describe a process or task and include:

- High-level flowcharts

- Detailed flowcharts

- Deployment flowcharts

- Opportunity flowcharts

Descriptions of each type of flowchart along with examples showing the workflow for a typical outpatient visit are provided below:

- **High-level flowchart**

    Typically used to provide an overview of a process; as a starting point for construction of a detailed flowchart; or to communicate information about a process to executives.

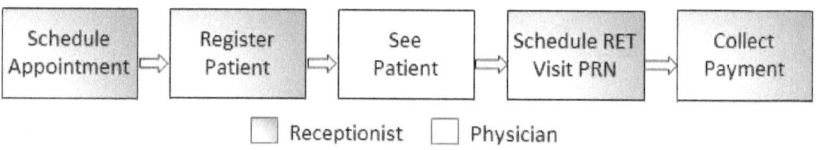

- **Detailed flowchart**

    Typically used to understand all steps in a process and how they're related; and to identify inefficiencies/redundant steps in a process.

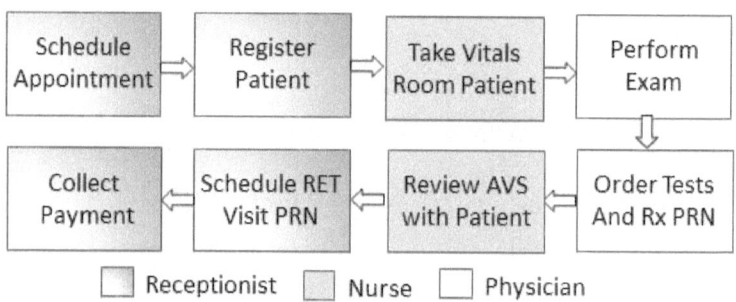

- **Deployment flowchart**

  Typically used to see how different positions/departments inter-relate to steps in a process; understand which positions and departments perform what tasks; and understand where handoffs occur.

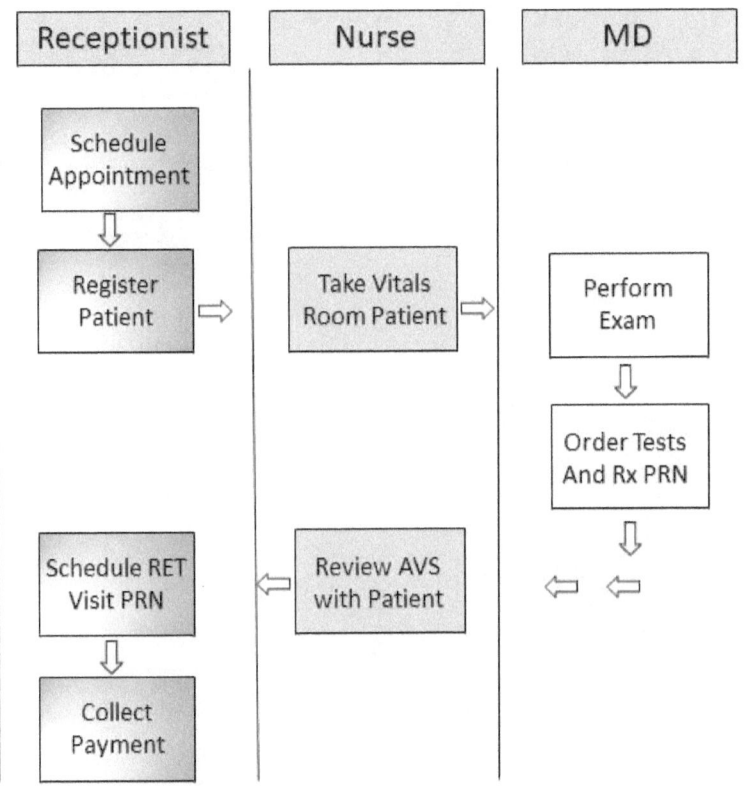

- ## **Opportunity flowchart**

  Typically used to identify and reduce "MUDA" or "waste".

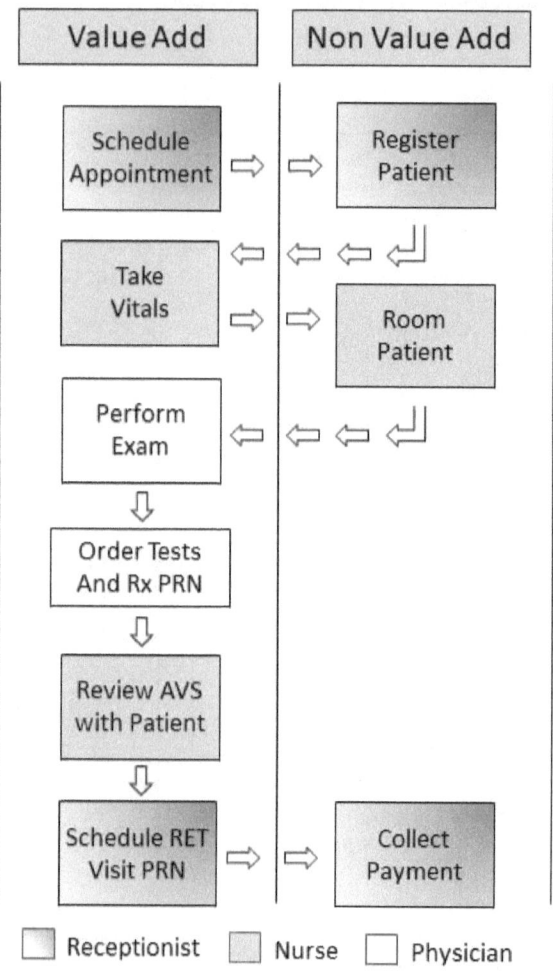

Once flowcharting of a task or process in your department or organization has been completed, review and evaluation are important to identify any opportunities for improvement or reduction of *"MUDA"* or "waste".

Opportunities for improvement can be identified by following the six (6) steps described below:

1. Review each step of the process or procedure

2. Identify any unnecessary steps *(i.e., steps that may not even have to be performed any longer because the need no longer exists)*

3. Identify any steps that are redundant *(i.e., steps that have already been performed elsewhere in the process)*

4. Identify any steps that can be changed or simplified *(i.e., steps that can actually be done differently or automated)*

5. Identify any steps that can be consolidated (*i.e., combining separate steps when possible into one step)*

6. Identify any steps where delays or backtracking can be reduced or eliminated *(i.e., reducing downtime between cycles by batching work)*

Most of the time, opportunities will be readily apparent from review of the flowchart or process map.

Sometimes, however, more information may be required to identify potential "waste" than may be provided by a flowchart or process map.

In those situations, a *value stream* map may be helpful in providing the information required to make the presence of *"MUDA"* or "waste" in your department or organization *visible*.

2.4   Value Stream Map

A *value stream* map is a visual representation of the key activities required to deliver a service or product to a customer (from start to finish).

One of the key differences between a flowchart or process map and a value stream map is the level of operational information provided.

Whereas a process map or flowchart just shows the sequence of steps and decisions involved in a process, a value stream map also includes key operational information, such as:

- **Cycle times**

  Cycle time is the time from when a task or operation begins to the point of time when the task or operation ends.

- **Set up or change over times**

  Time required to ready a device, machine, process, or system to function or accept a job. This is a subset of cycle time.

- **Wait time**

  The period or amount of time during which something is delayed.

- **Takt time**

  Takt time is the speed with which the product needs to be created in order to satisfy the needs of the customer and is calculated using the formula:

  $$\frac{Net\ Time\ Available\ for\ Production\ or\ Work}{Customer's\ Daily\ Demand}$$

- **Lead time**

  Lead time is the time from when a request is initiated until delivery of the product or service is completed.

- **Error or defect rates**

  The defect rate is a measure of the relative number of units that are defective or fail to meet prescribed specifications and is usually measured in terms of percent defective or defects per hundred, thousand, or million units.

- **Work in process**

  Work in process are a company's partially finished goods waiting for completion and eventual sale. These items are either just being fabricated or waiting for further processing in a queue or a buffer storage (in healthcare, work-in-process could be patients).

The layout of a value stream map is another key difference between a flowchart or process map and a value stream map.

A value stream map typically consists of three (3) sections that include:

- Information systems and flow

- Processes and data blocks

- Lead time and work time calculations

This information is typically laid out as shown on the following page in a generic value stream map.

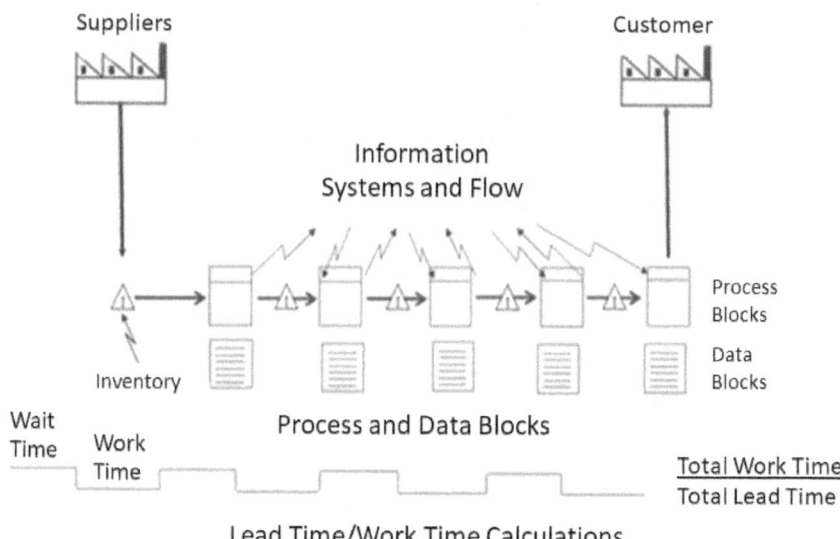

Lead Time/Work Time Calculations

An example of a value stream map for a *typical* outpatient visit is shown below:

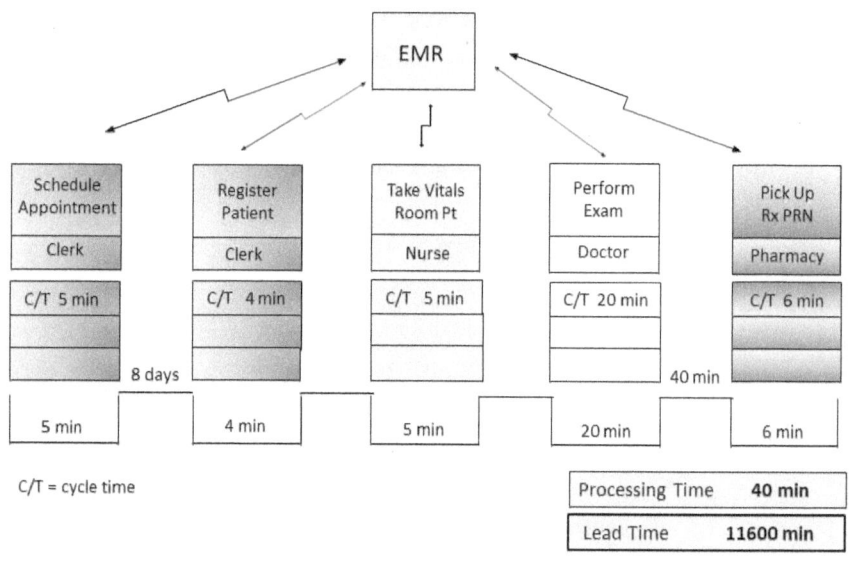

To construct a value stream map, follow the five (5) steps identified below:

1. Observe the process and information flows

2. Map the process flow

3. Add the information flows

4. Collect the required data and insert in the data blocks

5. Calculate the lead and work time and add to timeline

Occasionally, some of the information that may be needed to fill in the data blocks is not available; necessitating collection of the data required.

Most of the missing information may be obtained by using one (or more) of the following collection techniques:

- Observation

- Time study

- Work sampling

- Querying of available databases

- Manual check sheets

Once mapping of the key value streams in your department or organization has been completed, the map can be evaluated to identify any opportunities for improvement or reduction of "MUDA" or "waste".

Potential opportunities for improvement may be identified by:

1. Reviewing each step in the value stream

2. Identifying any steps or activities that do not add "value" from the customer's perspective *(i.e. a step or activity the customer would not be willing to pay for)*

3. Identifying any steps or activities that are not "capable" *(i.e. have a high error or defect rate)*

4. Identifying any steps or activities that are not "adequate" or "available" *(i.e. result in delays or wait for service, information, or materials)*

Looking at the value stream map below for a typical outpatient visit, several opportunities for reduction of "MUDA" can be *"seen"*.

These opportunities, see circled information, include 1. reducing the wait time between scheduling of the appointment and the appointment date and 2. reducing the wait time at the pharmacy.

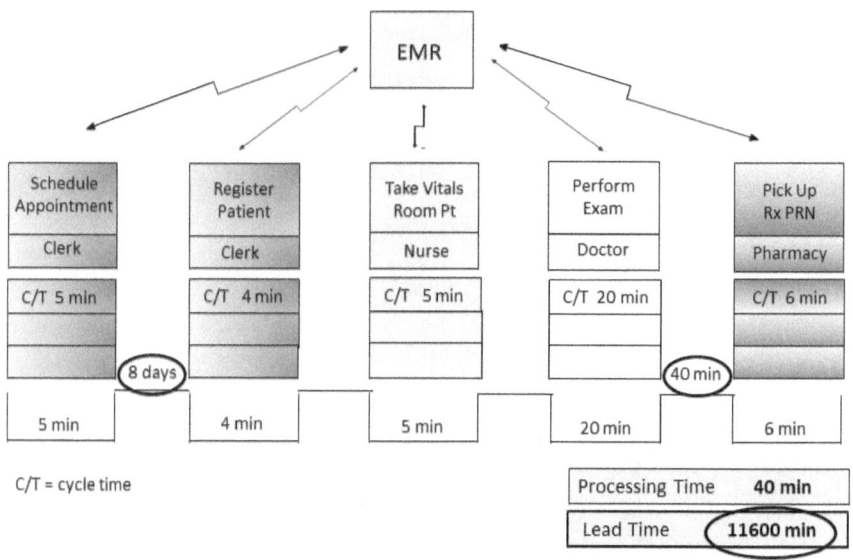

As can be seen, the key operational information incorporated into this value stream map makes opportunities for improvement more visible; facilitating the reduction or elimination of "*MUDA*" or "waste".

2.5   Benchmarking

Utilizing operational information can be helpful in making *"MUDA"* or "waste" *visible*.

Operational information typically includes:

- **Financial data**
  (i.e., cost data, profitability data, length of stay data, etc.)

- **Quality data**
  (i.e., infection rates, surgical complication rates, readmission rates, mortality rates, etc.)

- **Service data**
  (i.e., wait times, staff adherence to service standards, etc.)

- **Customer satisfaction data**
  (i.e., patient complaints, voluntary plan termination rates, patient survey results, etc.)

"MUDA" or "waste" can be made visible by *benchmarking* or comparing this information from your department or organization against that of similar areas within your company or industry.

The data needed for comparison of your department or organization against that of similar areas within your company or industry can be obtained from a number of different sources including:

- **Internal organizational databases**
  (i.e., financial database, EMR, quality database, etc.)

- **Industry support or trade organizations**
  (i.e., Institute for Healthcare Improvement, American Hospital Association, etc.)

- **Governmental agencies**
  (i.e., Centers for Medicare and Medicaid Services, Patient Advocate, etc.)

- **Benchmarking organizations**
  (i.e., iVantage Health Analytics, Premier, etc.)

A good example of how benchmarking can be used to make *"MUDA"* or "waste" *visible* is by looking at hospital readmission rates.

The data below compares the readmission rates for four hospitals with a diagnosis of COPD (culled from the CMS.gov website).

Hospital	Discharges	Predicted Readmit Rate	Expected Readmit Rate	Actual Discharges	Actual Discharge Rate
Hospital 1	291	18.4	19.9	48	16.4
Hospital 2	528	26.8	22.6	155	29.3
Hospital 3	139	19.3	19.5	26	18.7
Hospital 4	304	18.0	18.8	52	17.1

This data shows two readmission rates for each hospital:

- Predicted readmission rate
  This is the readmission rate based on the <u>specific</u> hospital's observed case mix and the hospital's effect on readmissions.

- Expected readmission rate
  This is the readmission rate based on the hospital's observed case mix and the <u>average</u> hospital's effect on readmissions.

In looking at the data for Hospital 2, a significant variance can be seen between the predicted and expected readmit rates; indicating an opportunity for improvement.

By reducing the hospital's readmission rate to the expected rate, the hospital could reduce readmissions by almost 16%.

The data also shows that Hospital 1 has a significantly lower readmission rate than would be expected based on its observed case mix; outperforming the three other hospitals included in the comparison.

By benchmarking and understanding the reasons for this outperformance, best practices may be identified that might be implemented in Hospital 2 to help lower their readmission rate for COPD patients.

Benchmarking has the ability, as demonstrated above, to help make opportunities that might not be *seen* with other approaches *visible*; helping to improve performance and reduce "*MUDA*" and "waste".

2.6   Variation

Measurement is an integral part of healthcare; with information being needed for the actual diagnosis and treatment of patients as well as the effective management of all the systems and processes required to provide the patient with care and services.

Some of the aspects of patient care and services that are routinely measured include:

- **Individual patient clinical information**
  (i.e., vital signs, lab results, etc.)

- **Clinical outcomes**
  (i.e., surgical complication rates, infection rates, etc.)

- **Process outcomes**
  (i.e., copay collection rates, denial rates, etc.)

- **Service**
  (i.e., patient satisfaction levels, patient wait times, etc.)

Significant variation in performance on many of these measures, however, is commonly seen both within and between similar departments and organizations.

These variances can stem from a number of different factors including:

- Differences in how staff and clinicians perform their work

- Differences in departmental or organizational policies, procedures, or practices

- Differences in staff and clinician skills, training, and knowledge

- Differences in the availability of the newest technologies

- The inherent randomness present in all processes

Such variation and its associated "waste" can often be made visible within a department or organization by using control charts.

A control chart (see example on next page) is simply a graph that represents data over time and shows how each data point relates to its average and to certain levels of standard deviation.

A control chart (see example on next page) typically has a center line which represents the data average/mean, an upper and lower control limit which typically represent 3 sigma or 3 standard deviations from the mean, and lines representing 1 and 2 sigma/standard deviations from the mean as necessary (not shown).

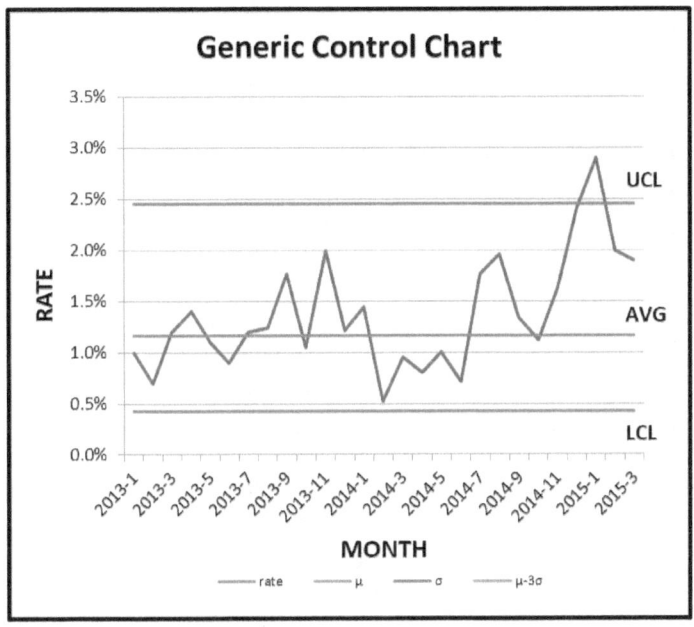

Where the data points fall on the graph relative to the average and these key levels (such as upper and lower control limits) can indicate the presence of "*MUDA*" or "waste" in a process.

When interpreting a control chart, the presence of certain patterns (see below) will tell you whether the variation is occurring due to special cause variation or common cause variation.

Pattern	Description
1	One of more points beyond the upper or lower control limits
2	2 out of 3 consecutive points in Zone A or beyond
3	4 out of 5 consecutive points in Zone B or beyond
4	7 or more consecutive points on one side of the central line
5	7 consecutive points trending up or trending down
6	8 consecutive points with no points in Zone C
7	15 consecutive points in Zone C
8	14 consecutive points alternating up and down

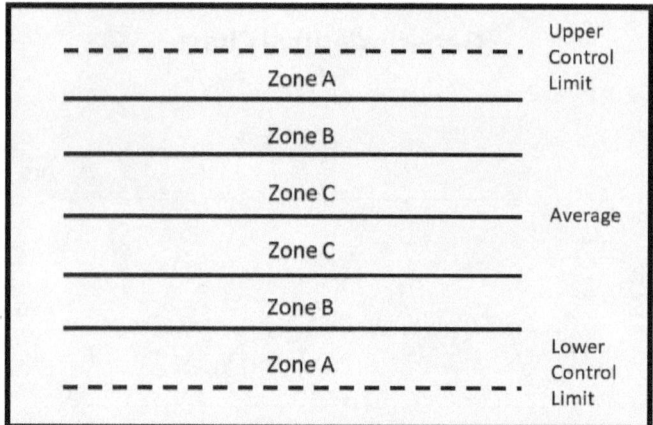

Special cause variation, defined by the patterns described on the previous page, is the result of a *specific* or *assignable* cause that can be identified and *acted upon* compared to common cause variation which is the result of inherent randomness present in the process.

An example of a control chart for vitrectomy rates, a procedure performed to address a complication associated with cataract surgery, is shown below:[10]

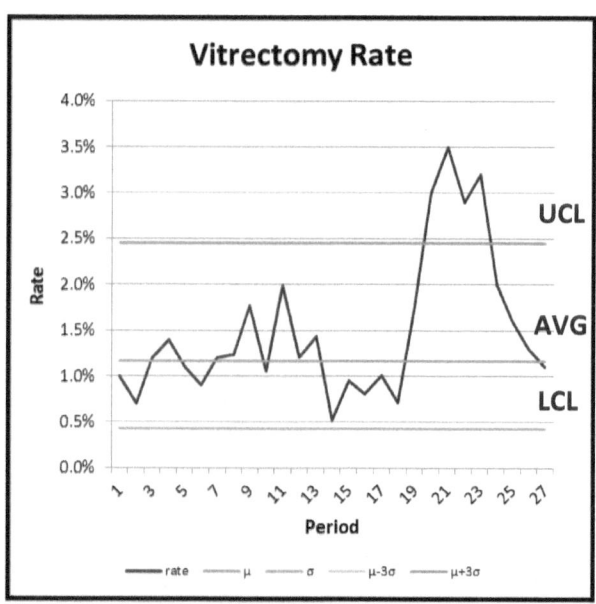

10. Based on actual data trends, events, and results experienced by the surgery center of one healthcare organization.

Looking at this control chart, the vitrectomy rates reported for periods 20 through 23 can be seen to exceed the upper control limit.

This indicates that something changed (special cause) starting in period 20 that increased the rate of vitrectomies that had to be performed.

What was found to have changed was the introduction of a volume based incentive program for the surgeons which encouraged some surgeons to stretch the limits of their efficiency; increasing the incidence of vitrectomies.

The incentive program was changed in period 24 to place a cap on the maximum number of cataracts that any surgeon could perform during a single surgical block.

After making this modification, the incidence of vitrectomies declined to earlier levels (see chart on previous page); demonstrating how control charts can help make potential "waste", along with the effectiveness of any actions taken, *visible* in a process.[10]

2.7   Customer Feedback

Most healthcare organizations receive some type of feedback about the service, care, or treatment they're providing to their patients or members.

This feedback, which may come from patient complaints, surveys, or focus groups, can help provide insight into *how* well a department or organization is performing.

Besides helping make *"MUDA"* or *"waste"* *visible*, such feedback can also help clarify what customers or patients *value*.

---

10. Based on actual data trends, events, and results experienced by the surgery center of one healthcare organization.

LEAN HEALTHCARE

To be useful, however, the raw data or feedback received from patients must first be organized in a way that is understandable, meaningful, and actionable.

A survey of patient satisfaction with outpatient appointment access was conducted by a large healthcare organization.

Data for this survey[11] was collected from over 5,000 patients and included patient feedback on:

- Whether the visit was scheduled for routine follow-up or an urgent problem

- Whether or not the patient had a personal care physician (PCP)

- Whether or not the patient saw their own personal care physician

- How satisfied the patient was with the number of days till they saw the physician

- How many days the patient estimated they waited from requesting the appointment till seeing the doctor

The data collected for *routine* appointments was summarized and showed:

1. An average patient satisfaction rating of 7 (out of a possible 10) which translated into patients generally being "satisfied" with the time they waited for their appointment

2. Only 43% of patients reported being highly satisfied (rating of 8 or above) with the time they waited for their appointment

11. Survey was a phone-based survey conducted by an independent organization unaffiliated with the healthcare organization being surveyed.

3. An average reported wait time of 15 days from the date the appointment was requested till the date of their appointment with the doctor

While these results indicated clear opportunities for improvement of both patient wait times and patient satisfaction, they did not however provide insight into what the patients *valued* and what they considered as a satisfactory wait time.

What the patients *valued*, however, was able to be inferred by correlating the wait times reported by each individual patient with the level of satisfaction they reported, and graphing the aggregated information.

Once graphed (see graph below), what patients valued became more *visible,* more *apparent,* and more *actionable*.

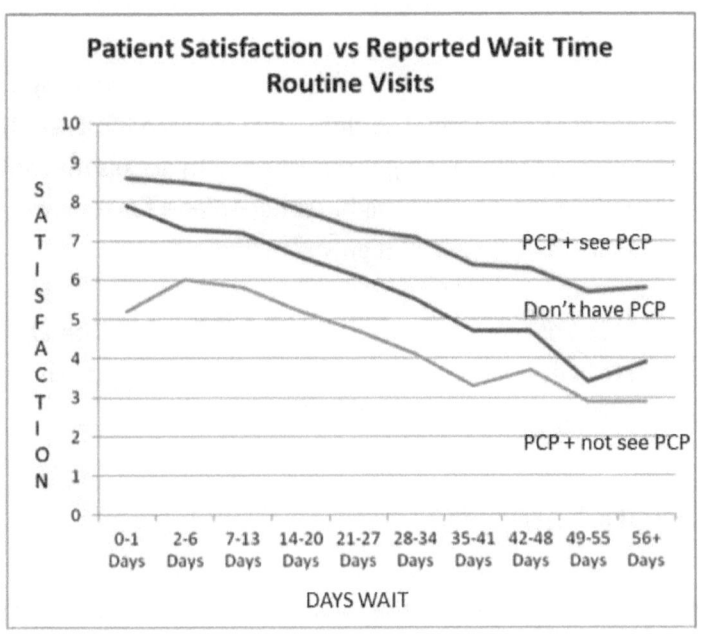

This graph clearly showed that patients *valued* seeing their own physician for *routine* visits and were <u>highly</u> satisfied even when they had to wait two weeks to be seen.

Patients, however, were merely satisfied if they had to see a physician other than their own personal physician for a *routine* visit even when the wait time was significantly less (within 0–6 days).

The data when graphed for urgent problems, however, showed the opposite.

According to that data, when patients had an urgent problem, patients *valued* speed over being able to see their own personal physician.

Patients were <u>highly</u> satisfied only if they could see their own doctor for an *urgent* problem within two days; otherwise most patients preferred being seen within two days by <u>any</u> doctor that was available.

This information was then used to revise appointment booking guidelines, which, along with other initiatives, helped increase the percent of patients that were <u>highly</u> satisfied with access for routine appointments from 43% to 81% highly satisfied and for urgent appointments from 41% to 83% highly satisfied.[12]

Customer or patient feedback can therefore not only be used to help identify "waste" within a department or organization, but can also be used to help identify what patients actually *value*.

2.8   Work Sampling

Staff and equipment are often the most expensive resources utilized in the delivery of healthcare.

12. Comparative results of survey conducted one year later.

It is therefore important to know how effectively these resources are being utilized.

Are they being focused on activities that provide "value" to the organization's patients?

Or are they sitting idle or being "wasted" on low priority tasks at the expense of more urgent activities?

One technique that can help identify whether these resources are being effectively utilized is work sampling.

Work sampling uses random observations of work activity to create a snapshot of the type and frequency of tasks that are being performed by staff or machines.

By taking these random observations, the proportion of time being spent on each activity can be estimated; helping make any "waste" or *"MUDA" visible*.

A random numbers table (see table on next page) or a random numbers generator are often used to determine when each observation should be made.

Numbers from this table can be translated into the times the observations are to be made by converting each random number into a minute equivalent (see appendix IV for how this is done).

RANDOM NUMBERS TABLE

63271	59986	71744	51102	15141	80714	58683	93108	13554	79945
88547	09896	95436	79115	08303	01041	20030	63754	08459	28364
55957	57243	83865	09911	19761	66535	40102	26646	60147	15702
46276	87453	44790	67122	45573	84358	21625	16999	13385	22782
55363	07449	34835	15290	76616	67191	12777	21861	68689	03263
69393	92785	49902	58447	42048	30378	87618	26933	40640	16281
13186	29431	88190	04588	38733	81290	89541	70290	40113	08243
17726	28652	56836	78351	47327	18518	92222	55201	27340	10493
36520	64465	05550	30157	82242	29520	69753	72602	23756	54935
81628	36100	39254	56835	37636	02421	98063	89641	64953	99337
84649	48968	75215	75498	49539	74240	03466	49292	36401	45525
63291	11618	12613	75055	43915	26488	41116	64531	56827	30825
70502	53225	03655	05915	37140	57051	48393	91322	25653	06543
06426	24771	59935	49801	11082	66762	94477	02494	88215	27191
20711	55609	29430	70165	45406	78484	31639	52009	18873	96927
41990	70538	77191	25860	55204	73417	83920	69468	74972	38712
72452	36618	76298	26678	89334	33938	95567	29380	75906	91807
37042	40318	57099	10528	09925	89773	41335	96244	29002	46453
53766	52875	15987	46962	67342	77592	57651	95508	80033	69828
90585	58955	53122	16025	84299	53310	67380	84249	25348	04332
32001	96293	37203	64516	51530	37069	40261	61374	05815	06714
62606	64324	46354	72157	67248	20135	49804	09226	64419	29457
10078	28073	85389	50324	14500	15562	64165	06125	71353	77669
91561	46145	24177	15294	10061	98124	75732	00815	83452	97355
13091	98112	53959	79607	52244	63303	10413	63839	74762	50289

The form shown on the next page can be used as a template for documenting each observation made.

This template can be preprinted with the most frequently performed activities and observations can be documented on the form using hash marks each time the activity is observed.

Any activities not preprinted on the form can be manually added to the task/activity column when observed.

LEAN HEALTHCARE

The number of observations that need to be made depends on the level of statistical accuracy needed (see appendix V for how to calculate sample size).

WORK SAMPLING OBSERVATION FORM

Position:													TOTAL	PERCENT	
Location:															
Date: DD/MM/YY															
TASK/ACTIVITY															

Total

However, sample sizes as small as 100 may be acceptable (despite what the sampling formula/table say) since the purpose of the sampling is just to identify potential "*MUDA*" or "waste" and not to set time standards, pay rates, or product costs which demand a higher level of accuracy and confidence.

Once the observations have been completed, the results can be tallied and reviewed for potential "*MUDA*" or "waste".

An example of a work sampling observation form for the non-RN staff in an ophthalmology clinic is shown on the next page.

This form was pre-printed with the most commonly performed activities for the six (6) medical assistants in the clinic.

A total of 101 observations were made of the activities performed by these medical assistants (see completed form below).

WORK SAMPLING OBSERVATION FORM

Position: Medical Assistant
Location: Ophthalmology Clinic
Date: DD/MM/YY

EMPLOYEE

TASK/ACTIVITY	Med Asst 1	Med Asst 2	Med Asst 3	Med Asst 4	Med Asst 5	Med Asst 6	TOTAL	PERCENT
Take vital signs	III	＋H	II	IIII	III	III	20	20%
Do visual acuity	II	III		I	III	II	11	11%
Search for items (i.e. supplies, equipment)		I	III	III	II	I	10	10%
Enter patient info in EMR	＋H II	IIII	＋H	III	III	III	25	25%
Review after visit summary with patient	II	I			II	II	7	7%
Review preop information with patient		II		I	II	II	7	7%
Stock exam room			I		II	II	5	5%
Answer phones	II	I	II			I	6	5%
Take messages for doctor	I		III	IIII		I	9	9%
Idle				I			1	1%
Total							101	100%

These observations showed that there was not much time wasted where staff were sitting idly with nothing to do (1%).

However, these observations did show that staff spent time on some activities that were considered unproductive and/or non-value-added.

Staff were found to have spent 10% of their time searching for needed equipment and/or supplies.

Reducing such "wasted" activity should be a priority and may be able to be recaptured by use of 5s (discussed in section 4.6 - Treating Motion Waste).

Besides spending 10% of their time searching for supplies and/or equipment, staff also spent almost a quarter of their time entering information into the patient's medical record (EMR).

Entering information into the medical record is considered an *essential*, but *non-value-added* activity.

Such necessary, but *non-value-added activity*, should also be minimized whenever possible.

Use of templates, smart phrases, and smart notes can reduce the amount of time required by staff to enter information into the medical record; helping to improve staff efficiency and productivity.

Work sampling can therefore help make the work activities of staff and/or machines *visible*; allowing actions to be taken that can reduce "waste" and improve performance.

2.9 Dynamic Modeling

All too often, the presence of "*MUDA*" or "waste" is identified only *after* a process or change has been implemented.

This is primarily due to the complexity of the systems and processes involved in the delivery of healthcare.

In many cases, however, potential "*MUDA*" or "waste" can be made visible *before* a process or change has even been implemented by using discrete event simulation.

Discrete event simulation uses computer software to dynamically model a business process so that the behavior of a process or system can be evaluated *before* the process or change has been implemented.

In many of the commercial products available, "blocks" are used to construct the process that is being modeled.

These "blocks" represent an action or activity that needs to occur during the process such as the arrival of a patient, the performance of a task, or the creation of a queue.

LEAN HEALTHCARE

Some of the most common blocks used[13] when modeling a business process include:

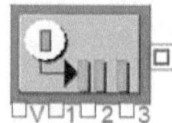

A generator block that creates items (i.e., patients, orders, etc.) at specified arrival rates (i.e., 10 minutes) for the simulation.

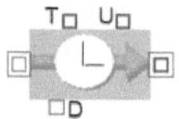

An activity block that holds a patient or unit of work for a specified processing period (i.e., 15 min per task) as well as provides utilization data for that block.

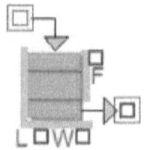

A queue block that acts as a buffer until another unit of work can progress to the next activity block as well as providing wait time data for units held in the block.

Values (i.e., interarrival rates, processing times, etc.) are entered into each block using a dialog box and the blocks are then connected together in the appropriate order to create the process that is to be modeled or simulated.

The simulation is then run; providing performance data such as wait times, lead times, and utilization rates that can help make potential "*MUDA*" or "waste" within the process *visible*.

An example of how simulation can be used in healthcare is demonstrated below for a laboratory that currently has six phlebotomy stations and an average patient wait time of 12 minutes (with some patients waiting over 40 minutes to have their blood drawn).

The laboratory wants to expand the number of phlebotomy draw stations but is uncertain whether it needs 7, 8, or 9 phlebotomy stations

13. The examples represent blocks used by Extend simulation software.

to ensure that none of their patients wait over 10 minutes to have their blood drawn.

A simulation model was constructed as shown below to find the minimum number of blood draw stations needed to meet their service target (no patient wait time over 10 minutes) while avoiding unnecessary construction costs ("waste").

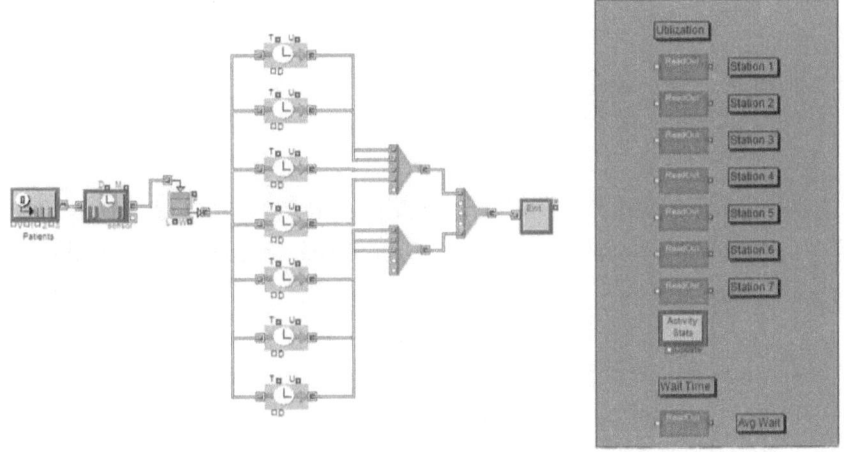

The model was built assuming that the blood draw time per patient averaged 5.5 minutes and that the patient arrival rate per hour (for the morning) averaged:

Time	Patient Volume
8 am – 9 am	70
9 am – 10 am	45
10 am – 11 am	80
11 am – noon	90
noon – 1 pm	30

The following results were obtained by running the model using these assumptions:

Measure	6 Stations	7 Stations	8 Stations	9 Stations
Avg Wait (min)	12	6	1.2	0.9
Max Wait (min)	41	27	9	7.5
Station Utilization	91%	86%	66%	60%

These results show that the maximum wait time can be reduced from over 40 minutes to 27 minutes by adding 1 additional blood draw station.

This wait time, however, still does not meet the service goal of having no patient wait of more than 10 minutes.

If, however, a second blood draw station is added (bringing the total to 8), the maximum wait time drops to 9 minutes which does meet the lab's service goal.

Therefore, a ninth station will not need to be constructed to meet the service goal for the current patient demand; thereby avoiding unnecessary construction costs or "waste".

Discrete event simulation can therefore help model the behavior of systems and processes and make potential "*MUDA*" or "waste" visible *before* any decisions have been made or actions taken.

DIAGNOSE

Identifying the Causes of Waste

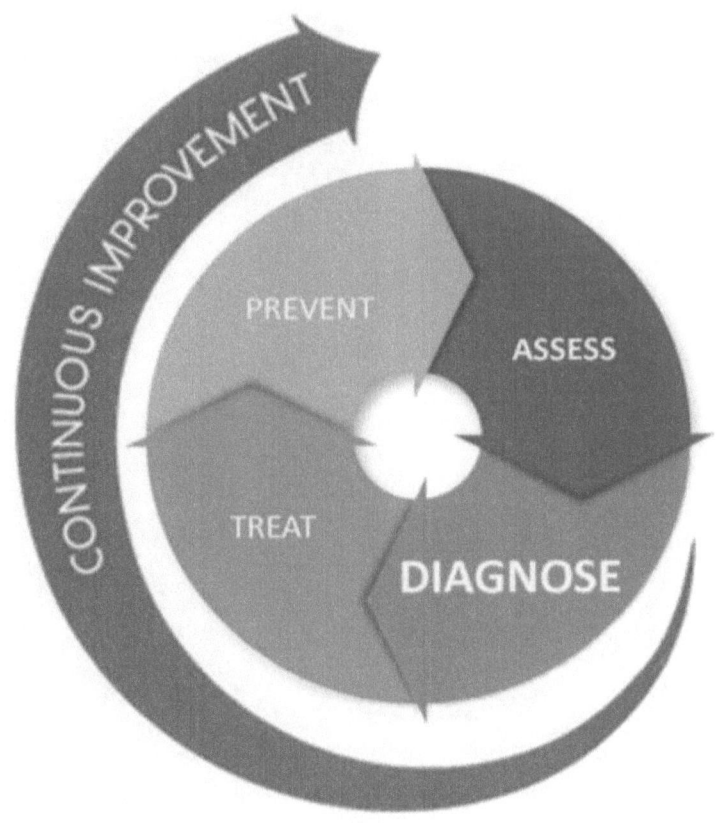

CHAPTER 3
How to Identify the Cause(s) of Waste

3.1   Now You See It

Identifying the presence of "waste" in a department or organization is important.

However, it is critical to understand what the underlying cause of the "waste" is before it can be reduced or eliminated.

Sometimes the cause of the "waste" is obvious and easy to "understand" such as when wait time for an appointment increases because a physician is out on an extended vacation or the number of surgeries decline because one operating room is temporarily closed for renovation.

At other times the cause of the "waste" can be more difficult to "diagnose" such as when wait time for an appointment increases because patients are being "churned" or the number of surgeries decline because of an increase in the number of last-minute cancellations.

So how can the cause(s) of "waste" in a department or organization be identified or "diagnosed"?

While a number of approaches are available to identify or "diagnose" the cause(s) of "waste" or "*MUDA*", there are three (3) tools/techniques that are most commonly used.

The widespread utilization of these three (3) approaches stem primarily from the ease with which they can be learned, the simplicity with which they can be applied, and their effectiveness in identifying the root cause of problems and include:

- the 5 WHYs

- the Fishbone diagram

- the Pareto diagram

3.2   Why? Why? Why? Why? Why?

Complex analytical tools are not always needed to "diagnose" the cause(s) of the "*MUDA*" or "waste" that have been identified in a department or organization.

Sometimes all that is needed is to ask just one simple question – "WHY?".

By repeatedly asking this one simple question it is often possible to drill down and determine what the root cause(s) are of any "*MUDA*" or "waste" that has been identified.

This iterative interrogative technique, called the 5 WHYs (see illustration on next page), depends on development of a clear description of the problem.

Once the problem has been clearly defined, ask "WHY?" using the answer to each subsequent response as the basis for the next question – until the "true" root cause has been identified.

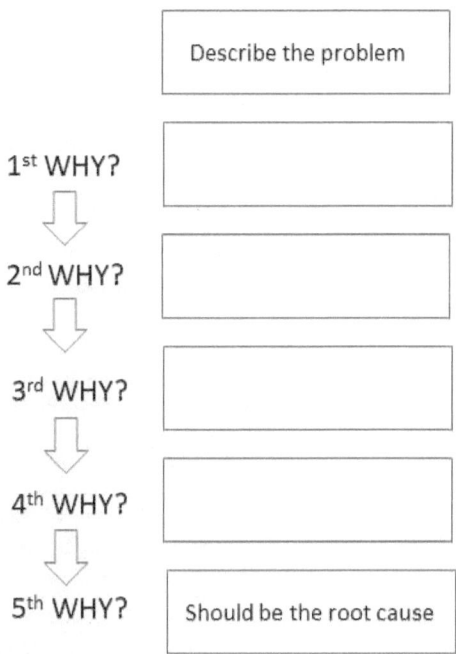

The example[14] on the next page shows how the 5 WHYs can be applied to "diagnose" the root cause of "waste" or "*MUDA*" in the operating room *(in this case the defect of a wrong hernia being removed)*:

In reviewing the case history, it was determined that:

1. The patient had multiple hernias

2. A pool physician had performed the actual surgical procedure

3. The initial consult had been performed by a different surgeon than the one that performed the surgery

14. The example is based on actual events that happened at one surgery center.

4. The pool surgeon had not seen the patient until the day of surgery

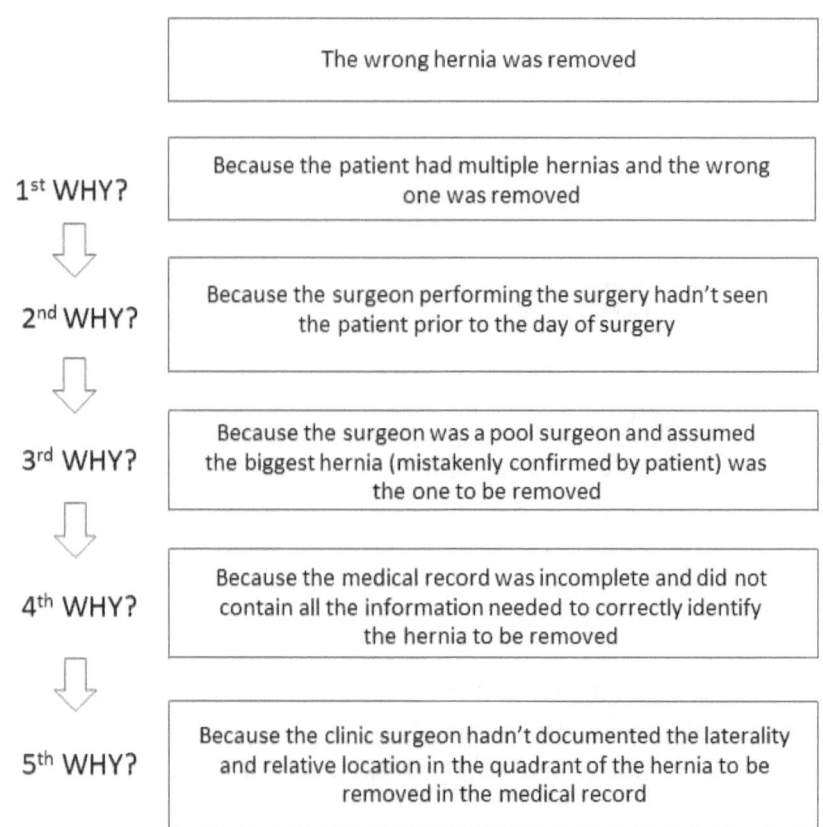

Initially most staff and clinicians thought that the use of a pool surgeon to perform the surgery was the *root cause* for the wrong hernia being removed.

However, after repeatedly drilling down by asking "WHY?" the *root cause* of the problem was identified and "diagnosed" to be a problem with the documentation in the medical record.

The staff and physicians concluded that the wrong hernia would not have been removed if the surgeon that initially saw the patient had documented the laterality and location in the quadrant of the hernia to be removed in the medical record.

The wrong hernia was therefore removed not because a pool surgeon had performed the surgery but because the documentation in the medical record had been deficient and incomplete.

This example demonstrates why it is important to:

- Involve staff and clinicians in conducting the analysis who are knowledgeable about the process or clinical situation

- Ask the correct questions

- Not confuse symptoms of the problem with the root cause of the problem

3.3   Fishbone Diagram

Another tool that can be used to "diagnose" the cause(s) of the "*MUDA*" or "waste" that have been identified in your department or organization is the FISHBONE diagram.

The fishbone diagram (see example next page) uses a visual approach to display and evaluate potential causes of "*MUDA*" or "waste".

The head of the fishbone diagram represents the problem, while the skeleton identifies the potential factors that are causing the problem.

Once the problem has clearly been identified, it is placed at the head of the fishbone diagram.

Potential cause "categories" are then identified and placed at the ends of

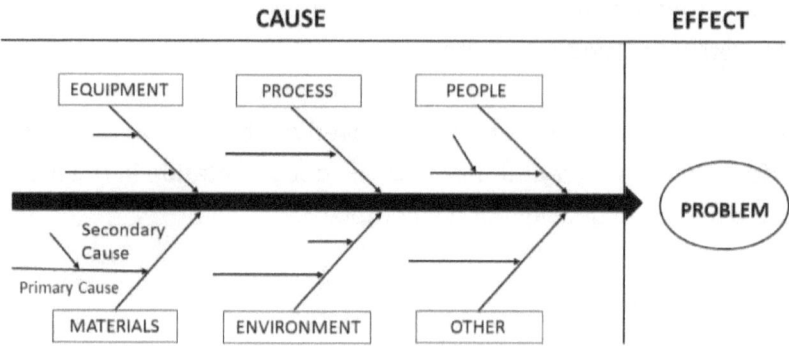

each rib to help guide the inquiry.

These "cause" categories are usually very broad in order to help stimulate inquiry and most commonly include:

- **The 3M's and P**
  Methods, Materials, Machinery, and People

- **The 4P's**
  Policies, Procedures, People, and Place

- **The 5Ws and 1H**
  What, Why, When, Where, Who, and How

- **The 6M's**
  Machine, Method, Materials, Measurement, Man and Mother Nature (Environment)

- **The 8P's**
  Price, Promotion, People, Processes, Place / Plant, Policies, Procedures & Product/Service

LEAN HEALTHCARE

Once the cause "categories" have been identified, an interrogative approach is used to drill down into each category looking for possible causes of the "*MUDA*" or "waste" that have been identified.

The potential causes identified are then further evaluated to determine which are the root cause(s) of the problem.

The example[15] below shows how the fishbone diagram can be applied to "diagnose" the root cause of "waste" or "MUDA" for a Family Practice Department *(in this case the defect of a high rate of patient DKAs or Did Not Keep Appointments)*:

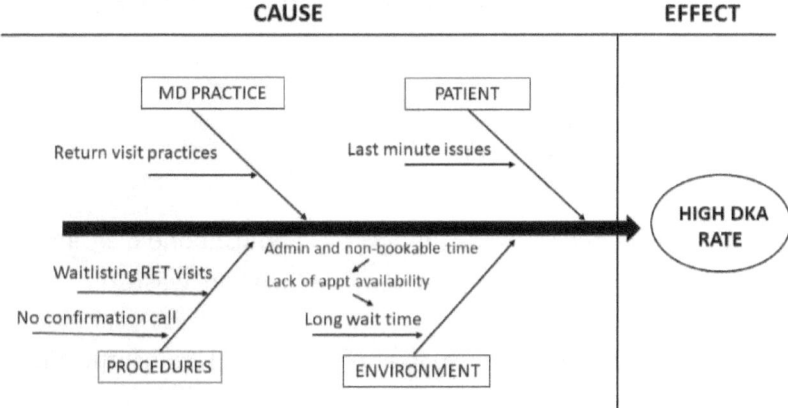

In this example the following four (4) broad categories were identified as potentially contributing to the high rate of DKAs:

- Procedures

- Physician Practice

- Patient (People)

- Environment

15. The example is based on actual issues experienced by a Family Practice Department with DKAs.

Drilling down into each category, a number of potential causes were identified for the high DKA rate ranging from long wait times for appointments to physician return visit practices to last minute patient issues.

After further evaluation it was determined that the *primary* cause for the high DKA rate was the long wait for appointments; the *secondary* cause being the lack of appointment availability; and the *root cause* being an excessive amount of administrative and non-bookable time on physician schedules.

Fishbone diagrams can therefore be a helpful tool for identifying or "diagnosing" the cause(s) of "*MUDA*" or "waste" in a department or organization.

3.4   Pareto Diagram

Interrogative techniques such as the 5 WHYs and fishbone diagrams can be helpful in "diagnosing" the cause(s) of "*MUDA*" or "waste".

However, there are times when such approaches will be insufficient to provide the insights needed.

Instead what will be needed to determine the cause(s) of "*MUDA*" or "waste" will be *actual* **DATA**.

The collection of such data may be accomplished *manually* using tally sheets, surveys, or observation; or *electronically* through queries of computer and electronic databases.

Once collected this data needs to be aggregated, organized, and displayed in a way that will be meaningful in order to be useful in identifying the cause(s) of "*MUDA*" or "waste".

The Pareto diagram (see below) is a tool that can help put the data collected into a meaningful and actionable format by arranging the various causal factors in *descending* order of magnitude.

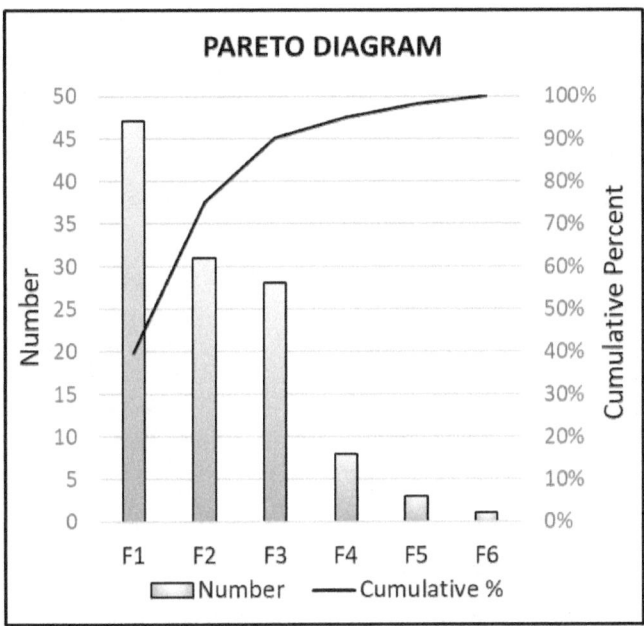

This ordering helps identify the "vital few" - the factors that warrant the most attention - from the "useful many" - factors that, while useful to know about, have a relatively smaller impact (see example on following page).

> *Note:* *According to the Pareto principle 80% of all effects or problems result from 20% of the causes (vital few).*

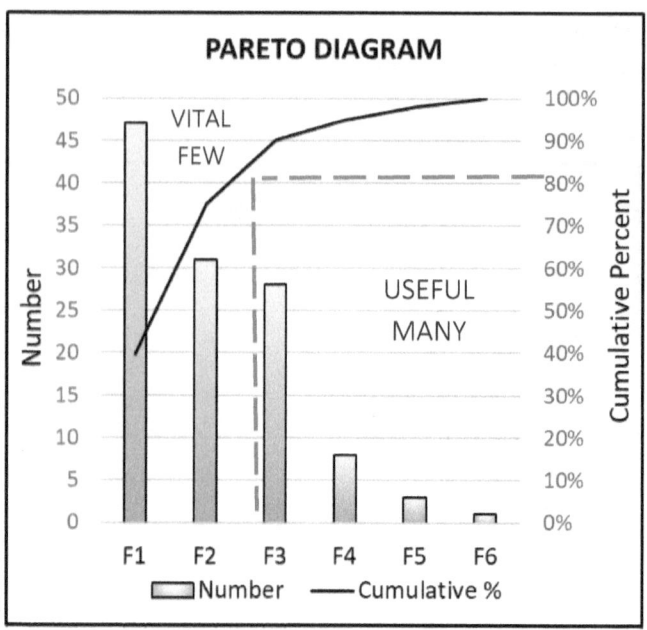

The number of occurrences for each causal factor are graphed as *bars* on the Pareto diagram while the cumulative percent is displayed as an *ascending line.*

An example[16] of how a Pareto chart can be constructed and used to identify potential *"MUDA"* or "waste" is shown below for the setup of instrument trays for surgical procedures performed in a hospital operating room.

The problems reported by staff and surgeons with the setup of instrument trays were tracked over time and then reported in the table on the following page.

16. The example is based on actual instrument tray issues reported by a hospital operating room.

Defect	Number	Percent
Damaged instrument (DI)	28	23.7%
Non functional instrument (NF)	8	6.8%
Wrong tray (WT)	3	2.5%
Missing instrument (MI)	31	26.3%
Wrong instrument (WI)	47	39.8%
Unsterile tray (UT)	1	0.9%
TOTAL	118	100%

Using this data as input, a Pareto diagram (see below) was created by

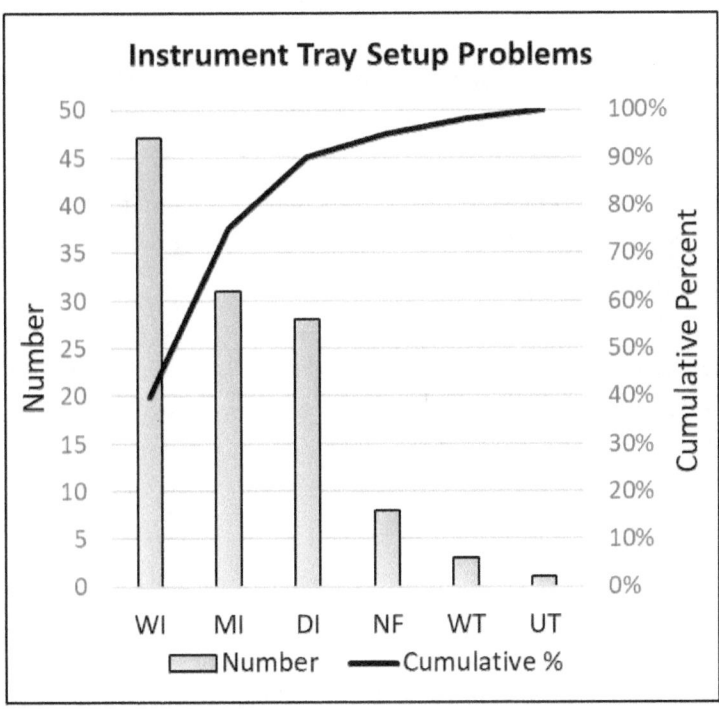

placing the defects in descending order of magnitude and adding a trendline for the cumulative percent.

Looking at this Pareto diagram, what stands out is that three issues –

damaged instruments, missing instruments, and wrong instruments – account for almost 90% of the problems reported.

By addressing just these three problem areas – the *vital few* – significant improvement in the quality of tray setup can be achieved.

Use of Pareto diagrams can therefore help highlight the main causes of "*MUDA*" or "waste" (in this case instrument tray defects); allowing improvement efforts to focus on the "vital few" rather than the "useful many".

3.5   Causes of "Waste"

Most departments and organizations differ significantly from one another in structure, function, and process.

Despite these differences, there is often significant similarity in the underlying causes of "*MUDA*" or "waste" found in most departments or organizations.

Some of the most common causes of "*MUDA*" found in healthcare are identified and described below for each of the eight (8) forms of "waste".

<u>DEFECTS</u>

Defects are one of the most important and high risk "wastes" that can occur in healthcare; sometimes with life threatening consequences.

Defects can range from incomplete or missing documentation and medication errors to misdiagnoses and wrong side/site surgeries.

Some of the most common causes of such DEFECTS include:

- Inadequate staff or clinician training or knowledge

- Lack of staff or clinician adherence to prescribed policies or procedures

- Poor, incomplete, or missing documentation

- Poor handoffs

- Technical failures (i.e., medical devices, implants, etc.)

- Inadequate staffing

WAITING

Waiting and delays for patients, providers, and staff is found throughout the entire healthcare system.

Waiting and delays can range from waiting for lab results and hospital beds to delays in when clinicians start making their rounds.

Some of the most common causes of such delays and WAITING include:

- Inadequate staffing

- Unbalanced workloads

- Poor scheduling practices

- Inconsistent clinician practice patterns

- Bottlenecks/lack of process flow/batching of work

- Poor handoffs

OVERPRODUCTION

Performing unnecessary tests, procedures, or activities can be very expensive...and in some cases even harmful to the patient.

Yet unnecessary or inappropriate diagnostic tests, surgeries, or admissions still happen at a concerning rate.

Why?

Some of the most common causes include:

- Efforts to maximize reimbursement

- Fear of malpractice claims

- Lack of clinician training or knowledge

- Patient demands for tests or procedures

TRANSPORTATION

A frequent complaint heard in healthcare is the unavailability of needed supplies, equipment, or beds.

The unavailability of these resources where needed results in the unnecessary movement of people, supplies, and equipment.

The unnecessary movement of these resources is entirely non-value added; contributing nothing to patient care or outcomes.

The need to move people, supplies, and equipment more frequently or further than necessary is often caused by:

- Poor facility or workstation design and layout

- Inadequate levels of supplies, equipment, or beds

- Poorly designed work processes or workflow (i.e., backtracking or unnecessary process steps)

- Poor scheduling, planning, or lack of coordination

MOTION

Wasted motion often translates into wasted energy, wasted effort, and wasted time.

Yet wasted motion is common in the delivery of healthcare - ranging from excessive walking to the performance of obsolete or unnecessary process steps.

Wasted or unnecessary motion, even when minimal, can result in costly inefficiencies especially when performed repeatedly over time.

Some of the most common causes of wasted motion include:

- Poor process or procedure design

- Poor workstation/facility design

- Isolated and/or siloed operations

- Lack of standards

OVERPROCESSING

Providing greater care or services than is required or expected by a customer or patient is often considered to be a competitive advantage.

Rather than being a benefit, however, overtreatment can actually result in harm to patients.

The reason that overtreatment can be harmful to patients is that it can expose them to unnecessary risk, potentially harmful side effects, as well as sometimes subjecting them to painful or debilitating procedures.

Some of the most common causes for overtreatment of patients include:

- Changes in technology which encourage treatment of even insignificant abnormalities

- Inappropriate or indiscriminate application of screening and/or treatment guidelines

- Minimizing the risk of potential liability (i.e., practicing defensive medicine)

- Maximizing reimbursement from third party payors

- Pressure from patients or family

INVENTORY

Inventory is a quantity or stock of items available for use in the delivery of healthcare.

The inventory may consist of:

- Medicines or supplies on hand in central distribution or on a nursing unit required for care and treatment of a patient

- Imaging equipment in the x-ray department or cardiac monitors on the intensive care unit used for diagnosing or monitoring a patient's clinical condition

- The supply of un-booked appointments on a physician schedule or the number of available/open beds on a nursing unit

While the nature of these inventories may differ, the causes of inventory "waste" are often similar and may include:

- Expiration of products, supplies, or services

- Overproduction or misallocation of services or over-purchasing of supplies

- Physician preferences forcing maintenance of similar products from different manufacturers in inventory

- Inadequate inventory management and control

HUMAN TALENT

Healthcare is heavily dependent on human talent to provide necessary care and services to patients.

Human talent represents one of the greatest expenses for most healthcare organizations.

Unutilized, underutilized, or inefficiently utilized staff or skills can therefore be a costly "waste".

Some of the most common causes of the "waste" of human talent include:

- Staff and workload imbalances

- Inefficient or out-dated processes

- Misallocation of resources

- Poor performing employees

- Ignoring staff input, suggestions, or feedback

Having identified the most common causes of "*MUDA*" for each of the eight (8) different forms of "waste" found in healthcare, what are the actions or steps that should be taken to "treat" or eliminate this "waste"?

TREAT

Eliminating Causes of Waste

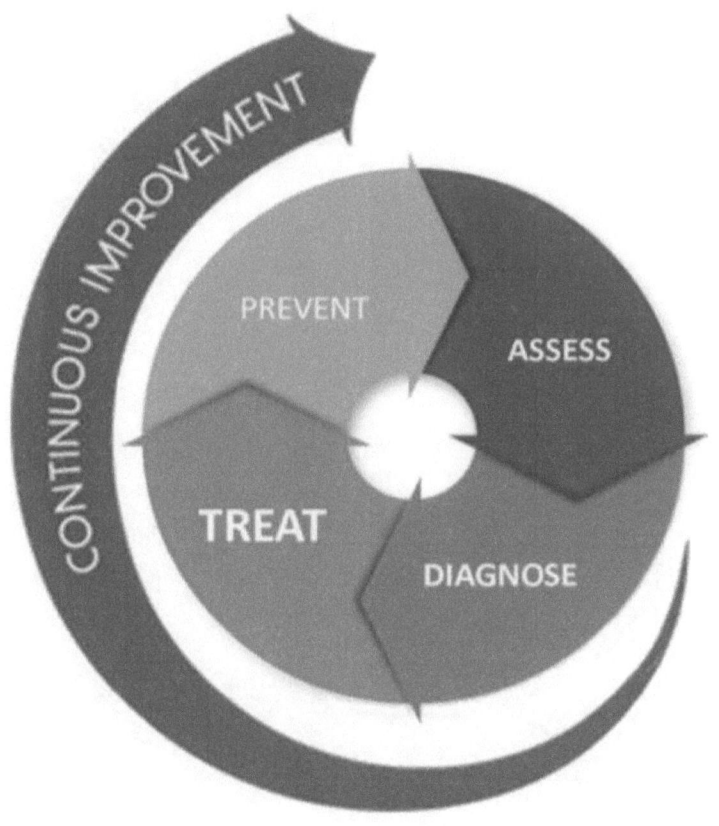

CHAPTER 4
How to Eliminate Cause(s) of Waste

4.1   What a Waste

Once a workup has been completed and the cause(s) of any *"MUDA"* diagnosed, it is time to develop a "treatment" plan to reduce or eliminate the underlying cause(s) of the identified "waste".

Sometimes the cause(s) of any identified "waste" are simple and can be quickly and easily "treated" (i.e., when a backlog for a diagnostic procedure develops due to a machine being down for repair or misinformation is given to a patient because a new employee misunderstood the policy or procedure).

At other times the cause(s) of the "waste" can be extremely challenging to "treat" (i.e., when a cluster of never events occurs in the surgical suite due to dissonance/communication problems within the team or lab utilization rates are high because clinicians can-not agree on ordering criteria).

While the actual issues specific to each department or organization will differ, many of the same strategies can be applied or tailored to "treat" each of the eight (8) different forms of "waste" which may be observed in a department or organization.

4.2 "Treating" DEFECT waste

Defects are one of the most important and high risk "wastes" that can occur in healthcare; sometimes with life-threatening consequences.

Besides causing serious harm to patients, defects in healthcare can also result in rework, increased costs, and even loss of revenue (i.e., Medicare not paying for the costs of preventable errors such as retrieval of retained foreign objects; treatment of bedsores, infections caused by prolonged use of urinary or vascular catheters, injuries from falls, etc.).

Defects occur in the delivery of healthcare for a number of reasons which range from inadequate process design to poor communication and handoffs.

Reducing or eliminating this type of "*MUDA*" or "waste" can require actions that involve avoiding reoccurrence of a defect and/or immediate detection and response to any defects which occur.

Some of the most common actions which can be taken to "treat" or reduce/eliminate defects include:

- Re-designing processes so they are less likely to produce re-occurrence of a defect (*Poka-Yoke*)

- Re-designing processes to detect abnormalities so they can be immediately corrected (*Jidoka*)

- Reducing or improving handoffs between staff, clinicians, and departments

- Implementing standardized work and/or checklists

- Reducing variation

- Utilizing new technologies

- Channeling

4.2.1 PROCESS REDESIGN (*Poka-Yoke*)

One way to eliminate defects is to "error proof" a process or procedure.

"Error" or "mistake" proofing involves re-designing processes so that a mistake can-**not** inadvertently be made by staff or clinicians due to either *physical*, *mechanical*, or *design* controls.

The types of controls typically used to "error proof" procedures include:

- Contact controls

- Fixed value controls

- Motion stop controls

Contact controls use physical shapes or sizes to prevent the use or connection of incorrect components to each other.

Some examples of *contact* controls utilized in healthcare include the use of different shaped connectors for hooking up medical devices to medical gases (i.e., square, round, octagonal, etc.), oral syringes designed so that they will not fit onto any IV tubing to avoid medication being administered intravenously, or defibrillator batteries that can only be inserted one way into the machine to ensure proper connectivity.

Fixed value controls use physical and visual methods to ensure that the correct quantity or criteria (i.e., weight, exposure level, etc.) required to meet specifications are adhered to.

Some examples of *fixed* value controls include devices that turn x-ray machines off whenever roentgen levels exceed acceptable levels, prepackaged surgical packs containing fixed quantities of supplies, or counting trays with a set number of holes for dispensing the right number of pills/medications.

The final type of control is *motion* controls which ensure that the correct number or sequence of steps have been followed.

Examples of *motion* controls include child proof bottles with twist caps that must be depressed and twisted before the cap can be removed, drive bars on portable x-ray machines which must be depressed and stay depressed in order for the unit to be moved, or wheel-chairs with automatic roll back systems which automatically lock the wheels when patients begin to stand up.

While incorporating mechanical, physical, or design controls into a process are the strongest approach for ensuring mistakes can-**not** inadvertently be made, not all processes or procedures are conducive to their use.

In those cases, procedural techniques are available which may minimize the risk of or allow immediate response to any errors or mistakes which occur.

4.2.2 PROCESS REDESIGN (*Jidoka*)

When mechanical or physical controls can-not be incorporated into a process or procedure to actually avoid an error from happening, then systems to warn of potential risk of error or mistake can be implemented.

One of the most common ways to warn of the potential risk of an error or mistake is to incorporate an *andon* into the design or redesign of the process or procedure.

An *andon* is a tool that signals a person or a team that there's an abnormality or defect in the process.

This *andon* can be a visual cue, an auditory cue, or a process or procedural cue.

The most important aspect of an *andon*, however, is not the light, the sound, or the tool, but rather the response to the *andon* which should be to immediately **STOP** the process and **TAKE ACTION** to address the cause of the error or mistake and restore the process to normal function.

Some common examples of *visual andons* in healthcare include lights on Code Blue carts to indicate they need to be checked for the day, computer screen alerts for pharmacists that warn of patient allergies or the presence of contraindications for prescribed medications, or a red light outside a room in a radiology suite indicating that caution needs to be exercised as imaging is in progress.

Common examples of *auditory andons* include the beeping on an infusion pump to signal that a medication is nearly gone or there is a problem with the tubing, the sound of a fire alarm warning of a possible fire, or the beeping of the bell from the annunciator panel in a Communications department alerting operators to the existence and location of a code blue.

The final type of alert is a process or *procedural andon*.

Procedural andons include timeouts which involve having a surgical team stop the process for a moment to confirm the patient's identity, procedure to be performed, and other critical information; sign-your-site procedures which require the surgeon to clearly mark the site of an invasive procedure with the patient looking on; or read-back where verbal orders received from a doctor are repeated back by the person receiving the order to ensure the accuracy of what has been heard.

The concept of any worker being able to "stop the line" has been a fundamental principle for ensuring quality in Toyota plants throughout the world.

Many operating rooms have adopted this concept using standardized language such as "I have a concern" which requires an immediate **STOP** to whatever is being done until the concern has been addressed.

A recent study showed that after adopting the universal protocol, which includes the use of timeouts, the incidence of wrong site surgeries dropped by almost 90% (from 0.16% to 0.02%).[17]

Incorporating physical, mechanical, design, or procedural controls into the design or redesign of a process are some of the most effective approaches for reducing or eliminating the "waste" of defects.

4.2.3 STANDARD WORK

Another way to reduce or eliminate defects is through the use of standard work.

Many errors or mistakes result from inconsistency in how a given process or procedure is performed by different staff and/or clinicians.

Applying the principles of "standard work" leads to increased consistency in the way a given task or process is performed by detailing the steps to be followed including:

17. Vachhani, J. & Klopfenstein, J. (2013). Incidence of neurosurgical wrong-site surgery before and after implementation of universal protocol. *Neurosurgery*:2013;72(4):590-5; discussion 595

- The precise **sequence** in which each step is to be performed

- The **cycle time, rate** (*TAKT* time), or **timeframe** each step must be completed in order to meet customer demand

- The standard **material** or **supplies** needed to complete each step or task

Visual aids, such as photographs or illustrations, may also be included as part of the standard work instructions to help staff and clinicians more easily understand and execute each step *(as 65% of people are visual learners and can process images more easily than text).*[18]

The lack of consistent handwashing or the use of improper handwashing techniques are significant problems in healthcare and major contributors to the high rate of hospital acquired infections.

The use of standard work can help increase consistency in *when* and *how* handwashing is performed; and reduce the incidence of hospital acquired infections (which affects 1 in 25 patients).[19]

The example on the next page for handwashing[20] shows how standard work can increase consistency in the way a given task is performed.

18. McCue, T. (2013). Why Infographics Rule. *Forbes*, Jan 8, 2013
https://www.forbes.com/sites/tjmccue/2013/01/08/what-is-an-infographic-and-ways-to-make-it-go-viral/#124721c27272

19. Clean Hands Count for Safe Healthcare, Center for Disease Control
https://www.cdc.gov/features/handhygiene/index.html

20. World Health Organization, Hand Hygiene: Why, How, and When brochure
https://www.who.int/gpsc/5may/Hand_Hygiene_Why_How_and_When_Brochure.pdf

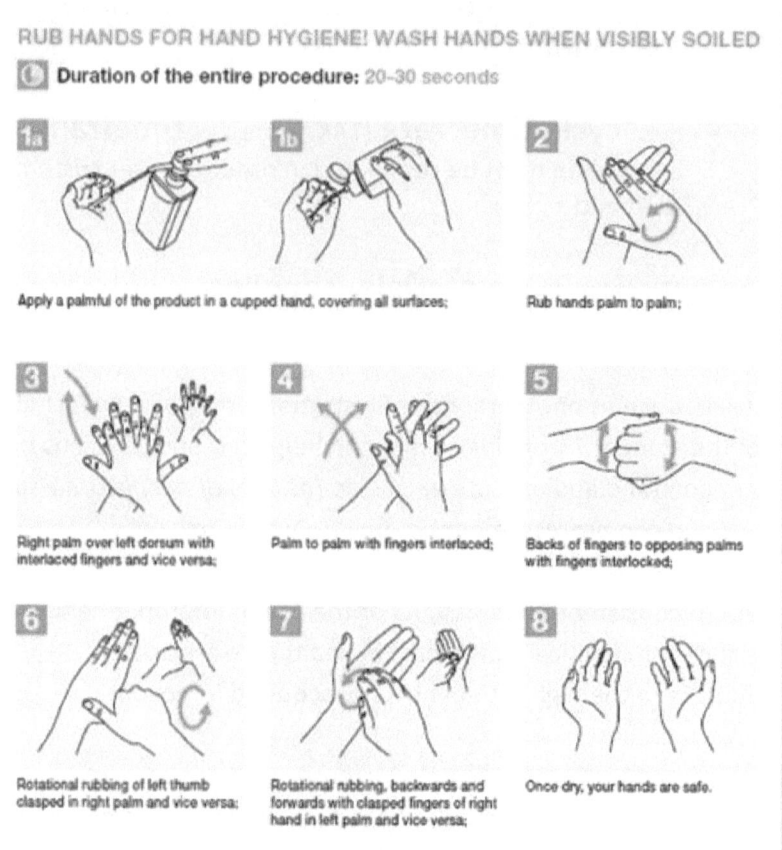

RUB HANDS FOR HAND HYGIENE! WASH HANDS WHEN VISIBLY SOILED

Duration of the entire procedure: 20-30 seconds

1a	1b	2
Apply a palmful of the product in a cupped hand, covering all surfaces;		Rub hands palm to palm;

3	4	5
Right palm over left dorsum with interlaced fingers and vice versa;	Palm to palm with fingers interlaced;	Backs of fingers to opposing palms with fingers interlocked;

6	7	8
Rotational rubbing of left thumb clasped in right palm and vice versa;	Rotational rubbing, backwards and forwards with clasped fingers of right hand in left palm and vice versa;	Once dry, your hands are safe.

Besides describing and illustrating the *steps* and *sequence* to be followed for hand washing, the standard work instruction sheet reminds employees and clinicians as to *when* they should wash their hands and for *how long*.

The CDC estimates that by increasing the consistency in when and how handwashing is performed, about 30% of diarrhea-related sicknesses and about 20% of respiratory infections (e.g., colds) could be prevented.[21]

Another example of standard work commonly used in healthcare is the

21. Show Me the Science – Why Wash Your Hands, Centers for Disease Control and Prevention
https://www.cdc.gov/handwashing/why-handwashing.html

clinical pathway.

A clinical pathway describes what actions the different staff and clinicians should take in the management of a patient for a specific clinical condition or diagnosis.

An example of a clinical pathway for embolic/thrombotic stroke is shown on the next page.

The clinical pathway not only describes what should be done, but also the sequence and timeframe in which these tasks and interventions should occur.

The effectiveness of using clinical pathways to reduce errors or mistakes was demonstrated in a study of patients undergoing total knee replacement.

Patients whose treatment was being managed using clinical pathways had 32% fewer adverse events than patients that were being managed in more traditional ways.[22]

In addition, the length of stay for these patients was shorter by 0.5 days, resulting in lower overall costs for the hospital and the patient.[22]

By applying the principles of standard work, consistency can be increased in *when* and *how* tasks are performed; helping to reduce the incidence of defects or errors that can affect the quality, safety, and affordability of patient care and services.

22. Husni et al. (2010). Decreasing medical complications for total knee arthroplasty: effect of critical pathways. *BMC Musculoskelet Disord.* 2010 Jul 14; 11():160. doi: 10.1186/1471-2474-11-160.
https://pubmed.ncbi.nlm.nih.gov/20630086/

Circle all that apply

	Day 1/Date:	Day 2/Date:	Day 3/Date:	Day 4/Date:	Day 5/Date:
Location	ED/Neuro Conc. Care/Floor	Neuro Conc. Care/Floor	Neuro Conc. Care/Floor	Neuro Conc. Care/Floor	Discharge
Admission/ Discharge	• Neuro Conc. Care • Telemetry • Assess for stroke study page 762-3549.	————————▶ • D/C coordinator eval.	Transfer to: • telemetry • floor	D/C plans finalized: • Home • Home/Home Health • Acute Rehab • Subacute care • SNF	D/C level of care: • Home • Home/Home Health • Acute Rehab • Subacute care • SNF
Tests	• CBC, PT, PTT • Renal Panel, CSP20 • ESR, CK • CT brain scan • CXR, EKG	• PTT prn heparin • Carotid Doppler • 2D echocardiogram • Transcranial doppler • MRI/MRA	• PTT prn heparin	• PTT prn heparin then DC • PT prn coumadin	• DC heparin ————————▶
Treatments	• VS/neuro assess. q 4hr Call MD for BP>180 syst. or >105 diast. • O2 prn • Daily weight prn	• VS/neuro assessment q 4hr ————————▶ • Evaluate telemetry	• VS/neuro assessment q 4hr ————————▶ • Evaluate telemetry	• VS/neuro assess. q 4hr ————————▶ • Evaluate Telemetry	• VS/neuro assess. q 4hr ————————▶ • DC telemetry
Fluids	• Normal saline IV • Saline loc	• Evaluate fluids	• Evaluate fluids	• Evaluate fluids	• DC fluids/saline loc
Medications	• Heparin 25,000U/250ml D5W w/Heparin protocol (check CT brain) • Enteric coated ASA prn • Meds as per home or MD order • Acetaminophen for T.>99	————————▶ • Coumadin prn • Ticlid prn • ASA prn	————————▶ • Coumadin prn • Ticlid prn • ASA prn	————————▶	• DC when desired range reached. ————————▶
Consults	• Cardiology prn • Neurology prn • Speech therapy • Occupational therapy • Physical therapy	• Speech/OT/PT prn • Dietary prn • Rehab evaluation	————————▶	• D/C	————————▶
Pt/Family ED	• Basic Stroke Binder • Education checklist	————————▶ • Videos	————————▶ • Coumadin booklet prn	————————▶	————————▶

4.2.4 HANDOFFS

Improving handoffs is another way to reduce or eliminate defects in healthcare.

A patient handoff, also referred to as transitioning, is the act of passing a patient and all pertinent information about that patient from one provider or caregiver to another.

According to the Joint Commission, communication problems account for almost 70% of sentinel events that occur in healthcare facilities[23]; with at least half of these being communication problems that take place during handoffs between caregivers.[24]

23. What's New in the Patient Safety World, Joint Commission Sentinel Event Alert on Handoffs, 10/17 https://www.patientsafetysolutions.com/docs/October_2017_Joint_Commission_Sentinel_Event_Alert_on_Handoffs.htm

24. Lee et al. (2016). Handoffs, safety culture, and practices: evidence from the hospital survey on patient safety culture. *BMC Health Serv Res*. 2016; 16: 254. doi: 10.1186/s12913-016-1502-7 https://www.ncbi.nlm.nih.gov/pmc/articles/PMC4941024/

Improving handoffs, which occur frequently between caregivers throughout the course of a patient's treatment, is therefore critical in reducing errors and mistakes in the delivery of patient care.

Some of the most common handoffs that occur during the course of a patient's treatment include:

- Patient handoffs between nurses at a shift change

- Patient handoffs between physicians when consultations are requested

- Patient handoffs when transitioning care between departments (i.e., after surgery between Anesthesiology and PACU)

- Patient handoffs when patients change levels of care (i.e., ICU to step-down unit)

- Patient handoffs when patients are transferred to nursing homes or discharged from the hospital to home health

Some of the ways that communication errors can be minimized during such handoffs include:

- Standardizing key elements, responsibilities, and language used during handoffs

- Incorporating read back or repeat back of handoff information and instructions into the handoff process

- Utilizing a structured tool such as a handoff checklist to validate that all critical information has been communicated

The use of SBAR is one approach increasingly being used in healthcare settings to prevent errors by standardizing the elements, format, and language used during patient handoffs.

SBAR is a simple pneumonic to remind staff and clinicians to cover the following critical elements when conducting their patient handoffs:

Situation (a concise statement of the problem)

Background (pertinent information related to the situation)

Assessment (analysis/considerations of options)

Recommendation (action requested/recommended)

When using SBAR, a clear and brief description of the **SITUATION** is provided.

Example: Patient X has several different prescriptions for drug Y, each with a different dosage.

Once the situation has been clearly described, additional **BACKGROUND** information related to the situation should be presented.

Example: Patient X is being treated for D disease and the dosages for drug Y that were prescribed are G mgs and T mgs.

The background information provided should be followed by an **ASSESSMENT** of the situation.

Example: Patient X is exhibiting the following symptoms at this time.

After providing an assessment, a **RECOMMENDATION** on what action to take should be offered.

Example: I think Patient X requires a dose of drug Y at this time. What dose of the medicine do you recommend?

This structured form of communication allows critical information to be conveyed between caregivers in a mutually recognized, concise format that can help minimize omission or misunderstanding of the information that needs to be conveyed.

The effectiveness of using SBAR for communication between caregivers has been demonstrated in numerous studies.

In one study, the number of incidents attributable to communication errors decreased by close to 70% following roll out of SBAR for communication during handoffs.[25]

Another technique commonly used for structuring the exchange of information between caregivers during handoffs is the *readback* or *repeat back*.

A *readback* or *repeat back* is a method for confirming that the information that was communicated to another person was correctly heard by the individual receiving the information.

This process, known by the mnemonic of the 4 Rs, consists of the following four (4) steps:

Relay (convey information or directions to another)

Repeat (repeat back what was heard)

Review (confirm information repeated back is accurate)

Reply (verbally acknowledge the accuracy of the information repeated back)

25. Randmaa et al. (2014). SBAR improves communication and safety climate and decreases incident reports due to communication errors in an anaesthetic clinic; a prospective study. *BMJ Open*, 2014:4

The *repeat back* process is initiated when one person relays or communicates information or directions to another.

   Example: Surgeon: "Nurse give me a 4-0 Vicryl on a PS-2".

The individual receiving the information then repeats back the information that they heard.

   Example: Nurse: "Okay, doctor, that was a 4-0 Vicryl on a PS-2".

The person who initially relayed the information or instructions then reviews the accuracy of the information repeated back and responds with the statement:

   Example: Surgeon: "Yes, that is correct".

or, if the information repeated back is incorrect:

   Example: Surgeon: "No, that is not correct".

and then repeats and reconfirms the *correct* information.

The use of the 4Rs during handoffs, as illustrated above, allows for any misunderstanding or misinterpretation of the information conveyed to be **immediately** caught and corrected; thereby minimizing the risk of any patient harm or injury.

The value of incorporating readbacks into critical communications was demonstrated by one organization which reduced its error rate for verbal orders from 9% to ZERO after requiring readbacks for all verbal orders.[26]

While SBAR and readbacks are effective for improving communication between individual caregivers, a different communication approach is

26. Verbal Orders, Read Back Protocol Can Reduce Error Rate to Zero, *MEDCG*, April 23, 2012
https://www.mdecg.com/verbal-orders-read-back-protocol-can-reduce-error-rate-to-zero/

required when handing off responsibility for care of a patient to an entire team (i.e., surgical team).

To avoid errors or mistakes, it is important that all members of the team have an understanding of critical information about the patient and their condition and how it relates to their role in caring for the patient.

One of the most effective ways for communicating important information about a patient to an entire team is by conducting a *briefing*.

A *briefing* is a quick meeting or *huddle* with all the members of a team with the purpose of gaining an understanding of a situation or sharing important information or concerns about next steps or actions to be taken.

Briefings prior to the start of surgery have now become a common practice in most operating rooms as a way to reduce adverse events (i.e., wrong side, wrong site, wrong procedure, wrong patient surgery).

These pre-op briefings typically include a review of the:

- Operative plan

- Patient risks

- Potential hazards

- Safety concerns

- Operating knowledge of required equipment

Many hospitals have identified which team members have primary accountability for sharing information during the briefing (see visual aid on next page) in order to ensure a smooth and comprehensive exchange of information.

Briefing Prior to Surgery

ENTIRE team present

Circulator	Surgeon
• Patient Name • Operation • Side of operation or incision • Other pertinent history or information	**Details of Surgery** • Type of operation, approach • Positioning • Equipment needed **Medications** • Prior to start of surgery • During surgery **Blood** • Units ordered • Blood type • Units available in OR • Transfusion equipment **Pathology** • Planned frozen section • Planned specimens **Fire Risk** • Risk level
Anesthesiologist	
• Type of anesthesia • Drug allergies • Antibiotic coverage	
Scrub	
• Instrument availability • Confirmation of instrument sterility	

By clearly defining *which* members of the team are responsible for sharing *what* information, the failure to communicate important information prior to the start of surgery is reduced; minimizing the risk of any harm or injury to the patient.

Studies have shown that when pre-operative briefings were conducted, miscommunication events were reduced by 53%.[27]

Besides a reduction in miscommunication events, preop briefings were also credited for an 80% reduction in surgical delays[28] and a 20% reduction in surgical morbidity.[29]

4.2.5 CHECKLISTS

The delivery of healthcare often involves complex processes and procedures; many of which involve steps which if missed or performed in the wrong order can result in serious harm to the patient.

One way to prevent the accidental omission or incorrect sequencing of any critical process step is through the use of a checklist.

A checklist is nothing more than a list of things to be checked or done and if necessary, the sequence in which those things are to be done.

To be effective a checklist should be short, simple, easy to read, and contain only the most critical information or actions to be taken.

Blood transfusions are complex and high-risk procedures that demand that certain tasks be completed to avoid complications or injury to patients.

Due to the serious risks associated with blood transfusions, many hospitals have developed checklists (see example on next page) to

27. Preoperative Briefing Improves Communication, Reduces Errors. *Science Daily*, May 27, 2009
https://www.sciencedaily.com/releases/2009/05/090526140743.htm

28. MacReady, N. (2014). OR Briefings Reduce Surgical Errors, Improve Outcomes. *Medscape*, July 11,2014
https://www.medscape.com/viewarticle/828127

29. Clemens, DR. (2014). OR Briefings Reduce Surgical Errors, Improve Outcomes. *Anesthesia Experts*,
August 19, 2014
https://anesthesiaexperts.com/uncategorized/briefings-reduce-surgical-errors-improve-outcomes/

ensure that all critical steps have been completed before beginning to transfuse a patient.

BLOOD TRANSFUSION PREADMINISTRATION BEDSIDE CHECKLIST

☐ **Verify patient identity**

☐ **Confirm this is the RIGHT patient for this transfusion**

☐ **Confirm RIGHT product**
(Rx, blood component label, patient compatibility label, component all match)

☐ **Confirm RIGHT pack**
(blood component label, patient compatibility labels match)

☐ **Confirm expiration date/time not passed**

☐ **Confirm integrity of pack**

At one hospital, the incidence of transfusion incidents was reduced from 0.3% to 0.1% following development and use of blood transfusion checklists and work instructions.[30]

Similar findings were found in the surgical setting where major complications were found to have declined by 36%, deaths by 47%, infections by 50%, and returns to the operating room by 25% following adoption of a preop checklist at several major hospitals.[31]

30. Shrivastava et al. (2016). Good Clinical Practices Toward Safe Transfusions: A Study of Blood Transfusion Process and Suggestions for Streamlining the Same. *International Journal of Research Foundation of Hospital & Healthcare Administration*, January-June 2016;4(1):1-4
https://pdfs.semanticscholar.org/5655/12817e07d28f681a2ebeca00ecabf72ab2fe.pdf

31. DeHeer, P. (2010). Why Your Hospital Should Be Using a Pre-op Checklist, *Podiatry Today*, April 22, 2010
https://www.podiatrytoday.com/blogged/why-your-hospital-should-be-using-a-pre-op-checklist

4.2.6 REDUCING VARIATION

Differences or *variation* in quality, cost, and outcomes are common in healthcare.

Such variation can frequently be seen not only between organizations, but also between individual providers.

While variation in healthcare is commonly measured in defects or errors per 100 or per thousand, in most industries variation is measured in defects per million; with a goal of six sigma or less than 3.4 defects per million.

One of the ways of eliminating "waste" or "*MUDA*" is by reducing the amount of variation in how healthcare is delivered; the primary objective of six sigma.

Such variation often occurs because of differences in physician training and practice; which can be addressed by trying to standardize the way care is being delivered.

A good example of how physician practice can impact clinical outcomes is the way total joint patients were managed at one hospital.

At this hospital, the average length of stay for total joint patients was found to be significantly shorter for one orthopedic surgeon than the other three joint surgeons; with no difference in clinical outcomes.

In trying to understand the reasons for the shorter length of stay it was determined that this surgeon used a different combination of pain medications than the other surgeons; allowing earlier mobilization and initiation of physical therapy for his patients.

After the findings were shared with the other surgeons, agreement was obtained to use this combination of pain medications for the management of all total joint patients.

The average length of stay for total joint patients dropped by 31% once a standardized approach to pain management was implemented and this variation in surgeon practice eliminated.[31A]

4.2.7 REDUCING PROCESS STEPS

Processes are often made up of a number of steps or activities.

During each step of a process, there exists the possibility for an error or mistake to occur; ranging from a simple transcription or transposition error to errors in critical thinking, judgement, or execution.

The probability that an error or defect will occur at any one step can vary widely which causes the defect rate for the entire process to equal the product of the error rates of each step in the process.

Therefore, in a three-step process with an error rate of 1% in each step the reliability of the entire system would be 97% and the total error rate for the process would be 3% (see calculations below).

Reliability   =   99% x 99% x 99%   = 97%

Error Rate   =   1 - (99% x 99% x 99%)   = 3%

The error rate for a two-step process exhibiting the same 1% error rate per step, however, would be only 2% (see calculations below).

Error Rate   =   1 - (99% x 99%)   = 2%

31A. Robertson et al. (2015). Implementation of an Accelerated Rehabilitation Protocol for Total Joint Arthroplasty in the Managed Care Setting: The Experience of One Institution. *Advances in Orthopedic Surgery*, Volume 2015, Article ID 387197 https://www.hindawi.com/journals/aos/2015/387197/

Therefore, the error rate can be reduced by decreasing the total number of steps in a process.

A good example of how reducing the number of process steps can impact the number of errors is by looking at a verbal order process, which is still quite common in healthcare.

When giving a verbal order, the physician tells the nurse or authorized individual what action to take such as to place an order for an x-ray.

The nurse or authorized individual would then document and place an order for the requested x-ray.

The order would typically be reviewed by a radiologist for appropriateness and the requested views taken by an x-ray tech.

The images would then be read and interpreted by the radiologist and a report dictated as illustrated in the flowchart on the next page.

An error can potentially occur at any of the steps shown in the flowchart.

These errors can include:

- Transcription or translation errors while taking or placing the verbal order

- Incorrect positioning or taking the wrong views while imaging the patient

- Missing abnormalities or misinterpretation of the images taken while reading the images

- Incorrect or missing information while transcribing the report.

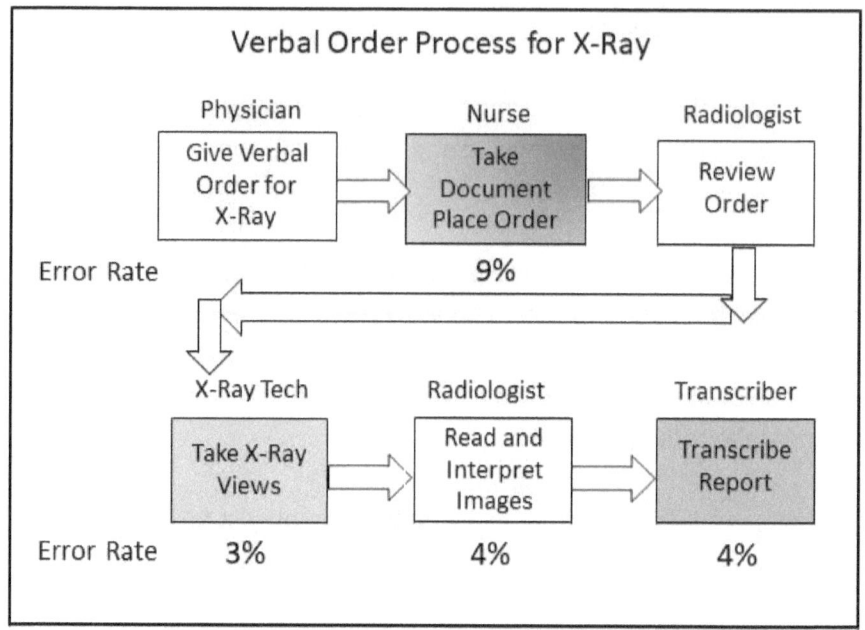

Assuming the error rates in the flowchart above[32, 33,34,35], the overall reliability of the process "R" would be estimated to average 81% (see calculation below).

R = (100% x 91% x 100% x 97% x 96% x 96%) = 81%

The probability of any one of these errors happening "F" during this

32. Verbal Orders, Read Back Protocol Can Reduce Error Rate to Zero. *MDECG*, April 23, 2012
www.mdecg.com/verbal-orders-read-back-protocol-can-reduce-error-rate-to-zero/

33. Doss, W. (2017). How to use simple checklists to decrease technologist error rates. *Radiology Business* May 30, 2017
https://www.radiologybusiness.com/topics/quality/how-use-simple-checklists-decrease-technologist-error-rates

34. Brady et al. (2012). Discrepancy and Error in Radiology: Concepts, Causes and Consequences. *Ulster Med J.* 2012 Jan; 81(1): 3–9, https://www.ncbi.nlm.nih.gov/pmc/articles/PMC3609674/

35. Lightfoote, J. (2011). Why I Prefer Transcription to Voice Recognition Software. *Diagnostic Imaging*, Nov 28, 2011, www.diagnosticimaging.com/blog/why-i-prefer-transcription-voice-recognition-software

process would then be estimated to average 19% (see calculation below).

F = 1 – (100% x 91% x 100% x 97% x 96% x 96%) = 19%

This process could be simplified by eliminating the verbal order step and requiring direct entry of the order by the physician (see below).

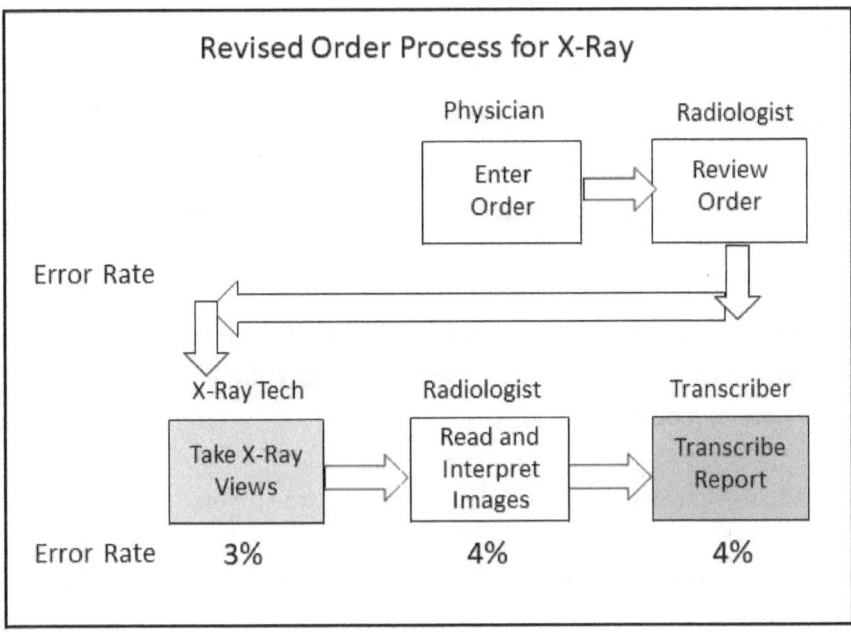

With this change in the process, the overall reliability of the process would be estimated to increase to 89% (see calculations below); resulting in an estimated 42% reduction in errors (see calculations below).

R = (100% x 100% x 97% x 96% x 96%) = 89%

F = 1 – (100% x 100% x 97% x 96% x 96%) = 11%

% reduction in errors = 1 – (0.11/ 0.19) = 42%

Similar results were found relative to medication administration.

Reductions of 40% - 55% in the number of medication errors were reported at several hospitals after implementing computerized physician order entry,[36, 37] further demonstrating how decreasing the complexity and number of steps in a process can significantly reduce the rate of errors or mistakes and improve patient safety and the quality of care provided.

4.2.8 USE OF TECHNOLOGY

Use of technology is another way to reduce or eliminate defects in healthcare.

A number of advances have been made in robotics and artificial intelligence (AI) which have had significant implications for how healthcare can be delivered.

A good example is the use of robots for prostate surgery.

Prostate surgery was traditionally done as an open or laparoscopic procedure.

This changed with the introduction of robots that can assist the surgeon during surgery.

The robot, which has articulated arms, performs the actual prostate surgery under the remote control of a surgeon who sits in front of a console in another part of the operating room.

36. Impact of Computerized Physician Order Entry on Medication Error Rates, Improvement Stories, Institute for Health Care Improvement
http://www.ihi.org/resources/Pages/ImprovementStories/ImpactofCPOEonMedicationErrorRate.aspx

37. Landrigan, C. & Friedman, J. (2007). Patient Safety and Medical Errors. *Comprehensive Pediatric Hospital Medicine*, 2007
https://www.sciencedirect.com/topics/medicine-and-dentistry/computerized-physician-order-entry

The robot, while mirroring the surgeon's hand movements, is able to filter out the minute tremors in the surgeon's hands which are often responsible for the inadvertent nicks or punctures that cause bleeding and infections commonly found with more traditional surgical techniques.

Besides providing the surgeon with greater stability in hand motions, the use of the robot also allows for smaller incisions and a magnified high definition 3D field of vision.

As a result, complication rates or "defects" normally associated with prostate surgery have significantly decreased.

PSA failure rates that are an early sign of biochemical progression and cancer recurrence have dropped from 20% for open procedures to less than 9% for robot assisted laparoscopic radical prostatectomies.[38]

In addition, the reported rate of positive surgical margins, which is another measure of treatment efficacy dropped from 35% for open prostatectomies to 15% for robot assisted laparoscopic radical prostatectomies.[38]

The use of robots and other forms of technology, as illustrated above, can help reduce the incidence of complications or errors; helping improve patient outcomes and the overall quality of care.

4.2.9 INSERVICING

Staff and clinicians are often required to have extensive clinical and/or technical knowledge and skills to successfully perform their jobs.

Defects or errors in the delivery of care or service sometimes result from

38. Finkelstein et al. (2010). Open Versus Laparoscopic Versus Robot-Assisted Laparoscopic Prostatectomy: The European and US Experience. *Rev Urol.* 2010 Winter; 12(1): 35–43
https://www.ncbi.nlm.nih.gov/pmc/articles/PMC2859140/

a misunderstanding of information, misapplication of policies and procedures, or lack of staff or clinician knowledge.

A good example of how inservicing can reduce defects or errors is the medical coding process.

Medical coding is important for medical record accuracy, governmental reporting, research, and financial reimbursement.

Data such as a patient's diagnosis and any procedures performed are abstracted from a patient's medical record and converted into 3-7 digit codes using coding systems such as the International Classification of Diseases (ICD) and/or the Current Procedural Terminology (CPT).

Use of these coding sets requires coders to have a detailed understanding of the diagnosis and procedure classification criteria and guidelines.

In one hospital, an audit identified that 30% of diagnoses and 25% of procedures were being coded incorrectly.[39]

Further analysis identified that the errors were the result of the coders using outdated or non-specific codes, incorrect modifiers, or failing to document laterality when required.

A plan was developed to in-service staff based on these findings.

Following this training, the error rate dropped to 4% for coding of diagnoses and less than 1% for coding of procedures;[39] demonstrating how inservicing can help maintain and/or improve staff or clinician skills and competency and reduce potential errors or mistakes.

39. Findings reflect results from a non-published study of coding accuracy pre and post inservice training in a community hospital.

4.2.10 CHANNELING

Expertise is developed from repetition and experience.

The more expertise a worker has, usually the better the work quality, results, and/or outcome.

This is particularly true in healthcare where clinicians may have to diagnose or treat obscure patient conditions or perform rarely or infrequently required surgeries or procedures.

A direct correlation has been shown between a clinicians' outcomes and the number of times they perform a particular surgery and/or treat a particular medical condition.[40]

By "channeling" selected patients to a limited number of clinicians, they acquire the volumes needed to develop the experience and expertise required to achieve these better outcomes.

A good example is the performance of radical prostatectomies.

One out of every nine men in the United States will be diagnosed with prostate cancer at some time during their life.[41]

The most common treatment for localized prostate cancer remains radical prostatectomy (RP) surgery which entails surgical removal of the entire prostate gland.

Most urologists (about 72%) perform radical prostatectomies as part of

40. Morche et al. (2016). Relationship between surgeon volume and outcomes: a systematic review of systematic reviews. Syst. Rev. 2016; 5: 204. published online Nov 29, 2016
https://www.ncbi.nlm.nih.gov/pmc/articles/PMC5129247/

41. Key Statistics for Prostate Cancer, American Cancer Society
https://www.cancer.org/cancer/prostate-cancer/about/key-statistics.html

their practice.[42]

However, the volume performed per year may vary significantly from surgeon to surgeon - with some urologists performing a low volume of this procedure and others a high volume.

Low-volume surgeons were defined in several studies as surgeons performing fewer than 40 radical prostatectomies per year and high-volume surgeons as performing 40 or more radical prostatectomies per year.[43]

The high-volume surgeons in these studies were found to have half the complication risk and shorter lengths of stay compared with the low-volume surgeons.[43]

Acquiring the minimum volume of patients or cases needed to develop expertise in management and treatment of certain patients or medical conditions is therefore critical.

Channeling or "directing" patients needing certain procedures to specific surgeons or specialists allows them to acquire the volume of cases needed to develop this expertise; and get better results and outcomes than if these patients were spread between all surgeons or physicians in a department.

The benefits of channeling, however, are not restricted to just surgery; as directing work to just a few individuals can help reduce the risk of errors or mistakes in any job that involves the performance of low volume or infrequently occurring tasks or activities.

42. Lowrance et al. (2012). Contemporary Open and Robotic Radical Prostatectomy Practice Patterns Among Urologists in the United States. *J Urol*. 2012 Jun; 187(6): 2087–2092
https://www.ncbi.nlm.nih.gov/pmc/articles/PMC3407038/

43. Hu et al. (2003). Role of Surgeon Volume in Radical Prostatectomy Outcomes. *Journal of Clinical Oncology* 21, no. 3 (February 1, 2003) 401-405. DOI: 10.1200/JCO.2003.05.169
https://ascopubs.org/doi/full/10.1200/JCO.2003.05.169

4.3 "Treating" WAITING waste

Waiting and delays are experienced by patients, providers, and staff throughout the entire healthcare system.

These delays can range from waiting for lab results to waiting for a hospital bed or surgery.

Besides resulting in high levels of dissatisfaction, waiting or delays can also result in rework, increased costs, and even potential harm or injury to patients.

Delays occur in the delivery of healthcare for a number of reasons ranging from inadequate staffing to inefficient procedures or workflow.

Reducing or eliminating this type of *"MUDA"* or "waste" can require actions that involve changes in physician practice, scheduling procedures, and/or utilization practices.

Some of the most common actions that can be taken to reduce or eliminate waiting time include:

- Shaping demand

- Redesigning processes and workflow to eliminate bottlenecks and create flow

- Reducing setup time and unplanned downtime

- Increasing capacity

- Implementing one-piece FLOW

4.3.1 SHAPING DEMAND

In many situations, waiting or delays are caused by an imbalance between supply and demand for appointments, beds, personnel, equipment, or some other limited resource.

When demand exceeds supply, waiting and delays go up.

As demand and supply come into balance, delays and the length of time patients, staff, or clinicians are required to wait goes down.

The goal is therefore to find the appropriate balance between supply and demand to minimize waiting or delays.

This can be achieved by either increasing capacity (supply) which often requires increased resources and cost or by shaping demand which often requires changes in patient, staff, or clinician behavior.

The changes in behavior involved in shaping demand are intended to either *shift* or *decrease* the number of patients, staff, or clinicians that are requesting care, service, or resources.

Some of the actions that can be taken to shape demand include:

- Load leveling

- Demand redistribution/shifting

- Demand reduction

Load Leveling

Heijunka (pronounced hi-JUNE-kuh) is a Japanese word that means "leveling".

LEAN HEALTHCARE

The principles of *heijunka* can be applied in healthcare to help balance and redistribute demand to reduce waiting and delays.

"MURA" and unevenness of demand can be found throughout the healthcare system from physician offices to hospital pharmacies and operating rooms.

Physician scheduling practices provide a good example of how the principles of *heijunka* can be applied to reduce patient wait times in the clinic on the day of their appointment.

Long patient waits in physician offices are common; with 40% of patients experiencing waits of 15 to 30 minutes in the waiting room and another 15% experiencing waits of 30 to 60 minutes before being seen according to recent studies.[44]

These long waits are one of the top complaints patients have with visiting their doctor,[45] and are often the direct result of physician scheduling practices.

One of the most common scheduling practices is for physicians to front load their schedule by booking several patients to arrive for their appointment at the same time.

Patients are typically frontloaded for either the first hour of each half day or every hour on the hour throughout the half day as illustrated in the examples on the next page.

44. McCormack, M. (2014). How to Treat Patient Wait-Time Woes. *Software Advice*, December 16, 2014
https://www.softwareadvice.com/resources/how-to-treat-patient-wait-time-woes/

45. Hitti, M. (2007). Waiting Room Tops Patient Complaints, Patients Generally Satisfied with Doctor-Patient Relationship, but Both Sides Have Gripes. WebMD, January 8, 2007
https://www.webmd.com/health-insurance/news/20070108/waiting-room-tops-patient-complaints

EXAMPLE
Frontloading of patients for the first hour of a half day

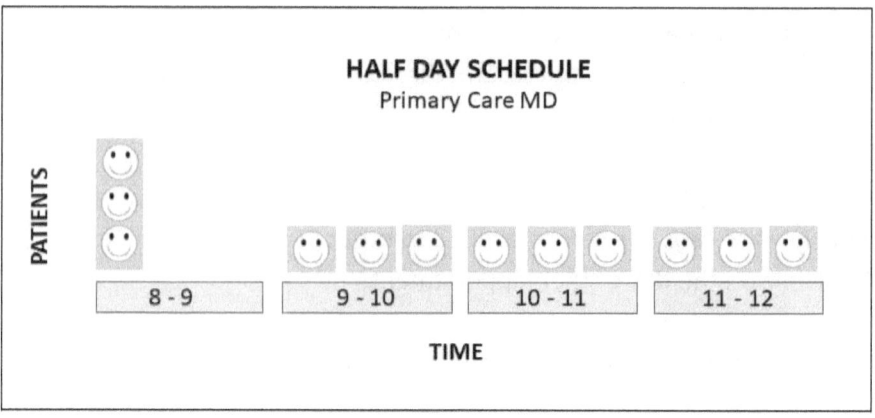

EXAMPLE
Frontloading of patients every hour on the hour throughout a half day

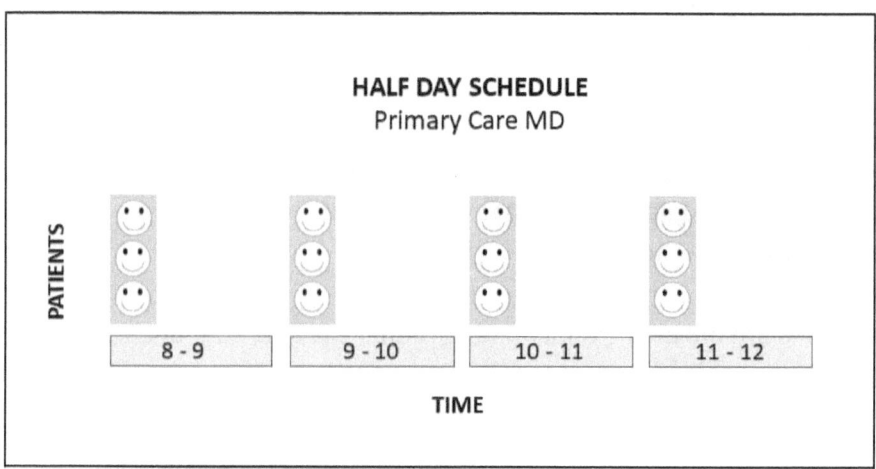

By frontloading their schedules in this way, physicians are able to optimize their time by maintaining a queue of patients.

This queue of patients reduces delays for the physician should one of their patients no show or arrive late.

While front loading helps reduce delays for the physician, it is done at the expense of patients that need to wait, resulting in delays, frustration, and dissatisfaction for them... the customer.

An analysis[46] of patient scheduling practices demonstrates how front loading of patients can impact patient wait times for a typical primary care clinic that schedules twelve (12) appointments per half day per physician and the physician being scheduled for an average of twenty (20) minutes to see each patient.

Frontloading	Average Wait (min)	Max Wait (min)	% Waiting	% Waiting > 30 min
First hour of half day	10	36	58	17
Every hour on the hour	23	48	75	33

As can be seen from the table above,[46] frontloading results in 17% to 33% of patients waiting greater than 30 minutes to see their physician; depending on which method of frontloading is used.

Rather than front loading the schedules as is often done by physicians, usually for their convenience; patients can be scheduled evenly, or load leveled, throughout the physician half day as illustrated on the next page.

By load leveling and eliminating "*MURA*" or unevenness in the scheduling of patients, patient wait times can be reduced by 70% to 90% (see table on next page) and wait times greater than 30 minutes totally eliminated; resulting in improved patient flow and increased patient satisfaction.[47]

46. Analysis based on results of discrete event simulation using Extend simulation software.

47. See appendix VI regarding the relationship between patient satisfaction and wait time in an MD office.

EXAMPLE
Level loading of patients per half day

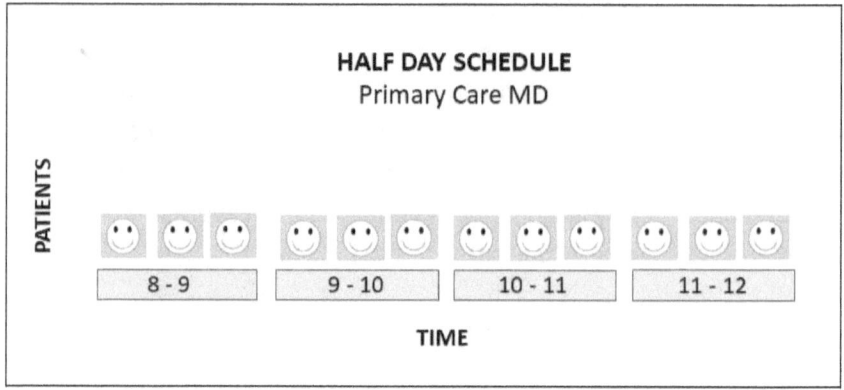

No Frontloading	Average Wait (min)	Max Wait (min)	% Waiting	% Waiting > 30 min
Evenly distributed	3	10	50	0

Shifting Demand

"*MURI*" is a Japanese word that means "overburdened".

When total demand exceeds total capacity, a worker or a system can become "overburdened".

Overburdening of workers, equipment, and processes is common throughout the healthcare system and results in many of the delays, bottlenecks, and dissatisfaction experienced by patients, staff, and clinicians.

When an entire system or process becomes overburdened, the principles of *heijunka* for balancing and eliminating "unevenness" will not be sufficient to reduce delays or waiting.

What will be needed instead are actions to shift or reduce total demand, thereby reducing "*MURI*" or overburdening.

Some of the most common strategies for influencing behavior in order to shift demand and reduce overburdening include the use of:

- **Pricing**
  (i.e., lower co-pay for urgent care versus emergency services to encourage use of urgent care for less serious medical problems)

- **Product or service substitution**
  (i.e., use of an NP or PA rather than a physician to see patients for certain types of appointments such as well baby appointments)

- **Timing or location**
  (i.e., free parking at an alternative location such as an outpatient clinic versus getting care at a medical center)

- **Education/Communication**
  (i.e., communicate to patients that they will have a shorter wait for services at certain times)

A simple example of how demand may be shifted is illustrated with the filling of prescriptions for an outpatient clinic pharmacy.

Prescriptions are often filled in an outpatient clinic pharmacy on a walk-in basis; often leading to long waits for the patients.

The wait times for a typical outpatient pharmacy with three (3) pharmacists, a demand of 73 patients for the pm half day with the volume distribution (see next page), and an average fill time of

11 minutes per prescription is shown in the table below.

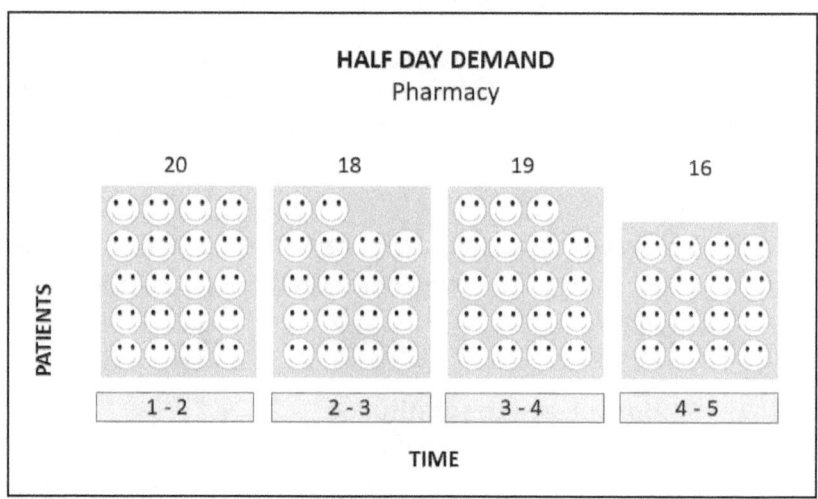

Average Wait (min)	Max Wait (min)	% Waiting = 11 min	% Waiting > 20 min
33	51	5	89

As can be seen from the table, patients would wait on average 33 minutes to have their prescription filled, with 89% of patients waiting over 20 minutes to receive their prescription.[48]

To handle this volume of prescriptions, the pharmacists must work a combined 2.7 hours of overtime to accommodate patients still in queue or in process at 5 pm.

The wait time for walk in patients could be reduced if some of this refill demand is shifted to mail-order delivery, which is also convenient for many patients.

If 10% of the prescription demand is shifted to a centralized mail-order

48. Analysis based on results of discrete event simulation using Extend simulation software.

location (see resulting distribution below), average patient wait times

HALF DAY DEMAND
Pharmacy

could be reduced by 39% and wait times greater than 20 minutes reduced by 46 percentage points (see table below) [49]; resulting in improved patient flow and increased patient satisfaction.

Average Wait (min)	Max Wait (min)	% Waiting = 11 min	% Waiting > 20 min
20	30	10	47

In addition, the amount of overtime worked by the pharmacists could be reduced from a combined 2.7 hours to a combined 12 minutes.

Since prescription demand was shifted but not eliminated, additional time to process the refill requests at the centralized mail-order facility is required; totaling 77 minutes for the 7 prescriptions now being filled at the mail-order facility.

The additional cost for overtime and processing of mail-order requests

49. Analysis based on results of discrete event simulation using Extend simulation software.

would total 1.6 hours of additional pay (12 minutes at 1.5 times plus 77 minutes for processing of mail order requests) compared to the 4.1 hours of additional pay if 10% of the demand had not been shifted to mail- order (2.7 hours overtime at 1.5 times).

The net effect of *shaping* demand by *shifting* a portion of the prescription volume to a centralized mail-order location is to reduce wait time for walk-in patients; while also achieving a slight reduction in total net cost.

Reducing Demand

Shifting of demand is one approach for addressing "*MURI*" or the "overburdening" of a process or system.

The downside to using this approach is that the work that has been shifted must be absorbed by the department or area that the work has been transferred to along with some or all of the associated costs.

"Overburdening" of a process or system can also be addressed by *reducing*, rather than merely *shifting*, demand.

Some of the most common strategies for influencing patient or clinician behavior is to actually reduce demand and reduce "overburdening" of processes or systems through the use of:

- **Pricing**
  (i.e., higher copays to reduce utilization or demand for services)

- **Order sets, clinical guidelines, and/or referral guidelines**
  (i.e., to standardize practices to reduce variation for referrals, treatments, return visits, ordering, admissions, discharges, etc.)

- **Incentives**
  (i.e., discount for low utilization of services)

- **Education**
  (i.e., reinforcing importance of taking, not running out of medicine)

A simple example of how demand may be reduced is illustrated by looking at provider return visit practices.

A common scheduling practice among optometrists is to bring patients back annually for routine vision checks even when there is no evidence or history of diabetes, high blood pressure, past vision problems, or the presence of other key risk factors.

This return visit practice can "overburden" the scheduling system; resulting in long patient waits for an appointment.

The wait times for a typical optometry clinic with five (5) optometrists, a patient demand of 435 appointments per week, of which 20% are annual return visits for patients without current vision problems or significant risk factors, with the volume distribution shown below and

WEEKLY DEMAND
Optometry

	Monday	Tuesday	Wednesday	Thursday	Friday
VISIT DEMAND	90	85	80	95	85

DAY OF WEEK

an average exam time of 30 minutes are shown in the table below.

Average Wait (days)	Max Wait (days)	% Waiting	% Waiting > 7 days
7	17	88	52

As can be seen from this table, patients would wait on average 7 days for their appointment; with some patients waiting up to 17 days, and 52% waiting greater than a week to be seen by the optometrist.[50]

The wait time for patients could be significantly reduced if some of this visit volume could be eliminated.

One way to reduce visit demand, and reduce "overburdening" of the system, is to change provider return visit practices.

Evidence-based studies have demonstrated that bringing back patients for annual vision exams who are asymptomatic and do not have current problems or risk factors is of limited clinical value and instead recommend bringing back patients:

- PRN when they have symptoms such as pink eye or

- When they experience a change in vision (i.e., blurry or double vision), or

- Based on evidence-based guidelines (such as those shown on the next page)[51]

50. Analysis based on results of discrete event simulation using Extend simulation software for 6-month period.

51 .Source: evidence based guidelines from Mayo Clinic and Kaiser Permanente
https://www.mayoclinic.org/tests-procedures/eye-exam/about/pac-20384655 and
https://healthy.kaiserpermanente.org/static/health-encyclopedia/en-us/kb/hw12/1865/hw121865.shtml

Age	Recommended Frequency If healthy and no vision problems
20 – 30	Every 5 -10 years
40 - 54	Every 2 - 4 years
55 - 64	Every 1 -3 years
65+	Every 1 - 2 years

By discontinuing the practice of scheduling routine annual vision exams for patients not meeting the recommended criteria, demand could be reduced by 20% with the remaining volume distributed as shown below; eliminating "*MURI*" and "overburdening" of the system.

WEEKLY DEMAND
Optometry

	Average Wait (days)	Max Wait (days)	% Waiting	% Waiting > 7 days

With this "unburdening" of the system, average patient wait times would be reduced by over 85% and wait times greater than a week totally eliminated (see table below) [52]; resulting in improved patient flow and greater provider and patient satisfaction.[53]

Average Wait (days)	Max Wait (days)	% Waiting	% Waiting > 7 days
1	1	0	0

52. Analysis based on results of discrete event simulation using Extend simulation software for 6-month period.

53. See appendix VII for statistics on patient satisfaction with appointment access.

4.3.2 REDESIGNING PROCESSES

Processes consist of a series of steps or tasks organized to provide patients with timely and appropriate care and services.

When these steps and tasks are well designed and coordinated, care and services "flow" without interruption or delay.

Bottlenecks or backlogs, however, can form when these steps and tasks are poorly designed, not integrated, of no added value, or dependent on outdated technology.

The development of these bottlenecks or backlogs can interrupt process "flow"; increasing cycle times and causing waits and delays for patients, staff, and clinicians.

Processes can be redesigned to eliminate the bottlenecks and backlogs that cause delays by applying the principles of work simplification.

These principles include:

- Eliminating unnecessary, redundant, or non-value-added steps

- Combining or rearranging steps whenever possible

- Performing steps in parallel rather than sequentially

- Reducing or eliminating changeover time

- Automating or mechanizing steps when possible

Eliminating Steps

Processes are made up of a number of steps or tasks.

Over time, as needs and technology change, some of these steps may become redundant, unnecessary, or of no added value (unless intentionally implemented as a barrier).

These steps however may remain a part of the process, causing inefficiencies and creating delays.

By eliminating these non-value-added steps and streamlining the process, waiting and delays can be reduced.

A classic example is the referral process for many specialty departments.

In many organizations, specialty doctors can only be seen by referral (often as a way to restrict access to limited, high-cost specialists).

In order to get a referral to a specialty department, the patient is required to be seen by their primary care provider.

The patient must therefore first wait to be seen by their primary care provider, get a referral, and then wait to be seen by the specialist.

This creates not only additional and often unnecessary delays, but also added costs (i.e., co-pays) for the patient, before the patient can be seen by the specialist.

In the example on the next page, a patient would wait a total of 26 days until they were actually able to see the dermatologist.

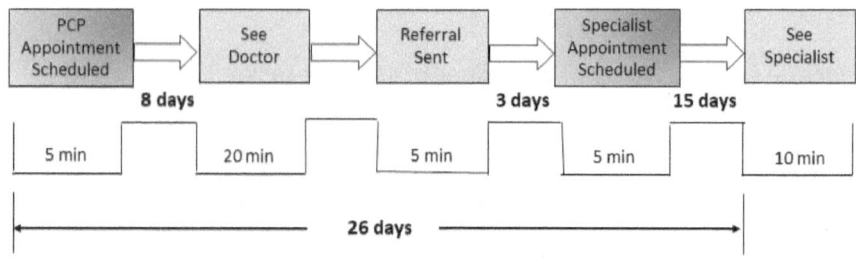

However, if the intermediate step of seeing the primary care provider could be eliminated for some or all of the patients by allowing self-referral or by using criteria-based guidelines, patient wait time (see below) would be reduced by 42% (from 26 days to 15 days).

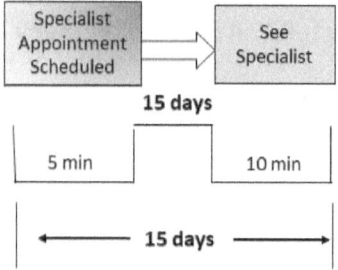

Besides significantly reducing patient wait times, eliminating the need for a referral would also reduce patient costs since patients would not have to pay the copay to see the primary care provider.

Combining or Rearranging Steps

Sometimes delays are not the result of the steps in a process, but rather the order in which those steps are performed.

If the order can be rearranged in which those steps are performed, it may be possible to avoid or reduce delays.

LEAN HEALTHCARE

A good example is the physical exam process.

Physical exams are typically performed on patients annually as a way to evaluate their overall medical status and pre-emptively identify and treat potential medical risks or issues.

The physical exam process typically consists of 4 steps that are performed in the following order:

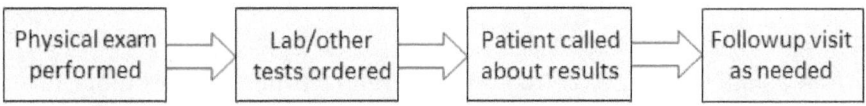

This sequence of steps results in test results not being available at the time of the visit; resulting in delay of potential discussions or decisions about potential issues or treatment decisions.

By rearranging the order of these steps and having the patient complete their lab/other tests prior to the visit (as shown in the diagram below), test results and potential issues or treatment options can be discussed during the physical exam rather than having to be delayed to some later date.

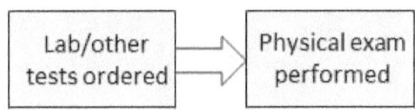

In addition, by eliminating the need for a follow-up call or visit, time is freed up for the doctor and additional co-payments avoided for the patient.

Performing Steps in Parallel

Tasks are typically organized in one of two ways - either sequentially or in parallel.

When tasks are organized sequentially or "in series", one task must be completed before the next task can begin.

This concept can be illustrated using the autopsy process.

When an autopsy is performed in a sequential order the pathologist performs the examination first and then writes or dictates their findings (see below).

Sequential Process

By organizing work in this manner, the next autopsy must wait until the findings have been dictated before it can be started.

Waiting or delays can be reduced if the tasks of a process can be performed in parallel.

Using the autopsy process as an example, the pathologist could dictate their findings in parallel as the examination is being performed (see diagram on next page).

Parallel Process

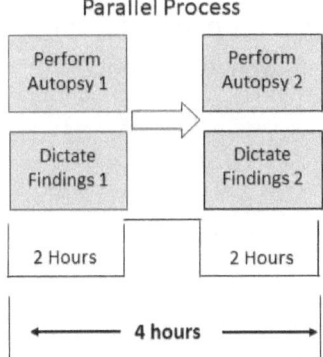

By performing the dictation in parallel with the exam, the time between the end of one exam and the start of the next can be reduced by the length of time required to complete the dictation; reducing delays and increasing throughput and capacity.

The principles of parallel processing can also be applied to processes involving more than one person.

A good example is the preparation of patients for surgery.

When preparing a patient for surgery many of the steps happen in parallel rather than in sequence.

A surgical team typically consists of a surgeon, a scrub, a circulator, and an anesthesiologist or CRNA.

While the circulator is "painting" or prepping the skin of the patient, the scrub is typically finishing unwrapping and setting up the instruments and disposables needed for the surgery, the surgeon is finishing scrubbing for the case, and the anesthesiologist or CRNA are managing the patient's vitals.

By working in parallel (i.e., at the same time) as shown below, the activities required to prepare a patient for surgery can be completed significantly faster than if done in sequence.

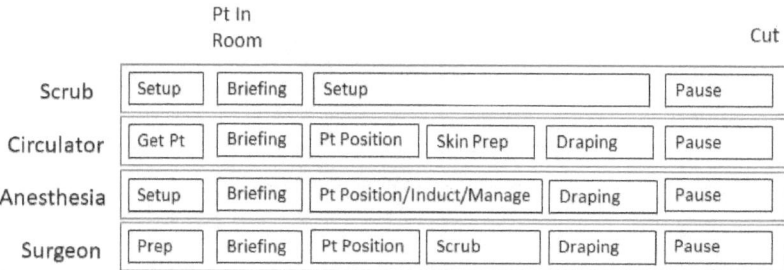

Automation/Use of Technology

Process redesign often involves the introduction of new technology into a process.

The use of technology can often reduce the cycle time needed to perform a task or activity, helping to minimize waits or delays.

A good example of how technology can help reduce the cycle time for healthcare processes is the use of autorefractors in optometry.

A typical vision examination takes 30 minutes and includes:

- Documentation of the patient's history

- Examination of the inside of the eye using a slit lamp to check the cornea, iris, lens, and the back of the eye, looking for signs of certain eye conditions

- Checking the patient's intraocular pressure using a tonometer

- Examination of the refractive status of the patient's eyes using a phoropter and lenses to determine the patient's prescriptive needs

An autorefractor is a machine that provides an objective measurement of a person's refractive error.

By using an **autorefractor** for the initial measurements rather than the traditional phoropter the time required for the subjective refraction test can be significantly reduced; allowing an optometrist to complete an exam in an average of 20 minutes rather than an average of 30 minutes.

The wait time for an appointment for an optometry clinic with five (5) optometrists, weekly patient demand of 435 patients, and an average appointment length of 30 minutes would average 7 days with some patients waiting up to 17 days, and 52% waiting greater than a week to be seen by the optometrist[54] as seen below:

Average Wait (days)	Max Wait (days)	% Waiting	% Waiting > 7 days
7	17	88	52

By incorporating the use of an autorefractor into the exam process, the length of time the optometrist must spend with a patient would be able to be reduced from 30 minutes to 20 minutes.

The impact of using this technology is that each optometrist would be able to see 8 more visits per day; reducing the average wait time for an appointment from 7 days to less than a day.[54]

54. Analysis based on results of discrete event simulation using Extend simulation software for 6-month period.

4.3.3 REDUCING CHANGEOVER TIME/SMED

Many processes in healthcare require time between tasks for setup or cleanup (changeover) before the next task can be performed or the next patient can be processed.

The time required for changeover is non-value added and delays the start of the next value-added step in the process and can typically be reduced by:

- Converting internal tasks for setup and/or cleanup to external tasks (as illustrated in diagram below)

   Internal tasks consist of those activities that must be performed while a machine or process is stopped whereas external tasks can be performed elsewhere and/or while a machine or activity is in process.

- Streamlining or eliminating internal or external tasks for setup and/or cleanup

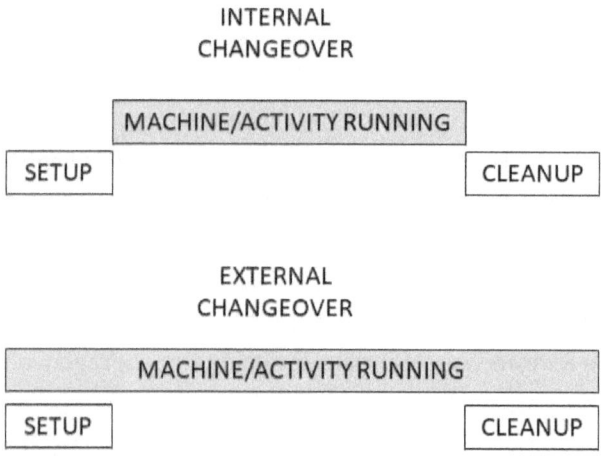

INTERNAL
CHANGEOVER

MACHINE/ACTIVITY RUNNING	
SETUP	CLEANUP

EXTERNAL
CHANGEOVER

MACHINE/ACTIVITY RUNNING	
SETUP	CLEANUP

A good example of how "internal" setup can be converted to "external"

See appendix VIII for more information on SMED.

setup to reduce changeover time is by looking at the computed tomography (CT) process implemented in the Imaging department at one hospital.

Computed tomography (CT) is a noninvasive diagnostic procedure which digitally combines multiple images taken from a rotating source into cross sectional images commonly called "slices" of the bones, blood vessels, and soft tissue inside the body.

CT scans are ordered for many reasons, including to:

- Diagnose muscle and bone disorders, such as bone tumors and fractures

- Pinpoint the location of a tumor, infection or blood clot

- Guide procedures such as surgery, biopsy and radiation therapy

- Detect and monitor diseases and conditions such as cancer, heart disease, lung nodules and liver masses

- Monitor the effectiveness of certain treatments, such as cancer treatment

- Detect internal injuries and internal bleeding

The practice in the CT department at this hospital was for patients to be given instructions and their cannula inserted (if necessary) while lying in the CT; resulting in the CT sitting idle while these activities were being performed.

After determining that these "internal" activities didn't actually need to be performed in the CT, but could be performed elsewhere, a room adjacent to the CT was identified.

This room was converted to a prep room where these activities were done; thereby converting these activities from "internal" to "external" tasks.

By freeing up the CT, another tech was then able to scan a different patient while these "changeover" activities were happening in the prep room; reducing the in-room time per study by 50% and recapturing enough time to scan six (6) additional patients per day.[55]

The increase in capacity resulted in a drop in wait times for exams; with patient wait times declining almost 70% (from an average 12 weeks to an average 4 weeks).[55]

Changeover time can also be reduced by *streamlining* the setup and/or cleanup process.

Room turnover in the operating room provides another good example of how a changeover process can be streamlined.

Upon completion of any surgery, the surgical suite must be cleaned and set up before the next surgery can begin.

This turnover process involves a number of tasks that must be completed before the next patient can be brought into the operating room such as:

- Tearing down the back-instrument table and mayo stand

- Gathering and removing all instruments and instrument trays

- Discarding and removing all disposable linens, supplies, and trash

55. Karstoft, J. & Tarp, L. (2011). Is Lean Management Implementable in a Department of Radiology? *Insights Imaging*. 2011 Jun; 2(3): 267–273
https://www.ncbi.nlm.nih.gov/pmc/articles/PMC3288997/

- Removing or wiping down dirty equipment

- Wiping down the surgical table and mopping the floor

- Wiping down all counters and surfaces with appropriate disinfectant

- Erasing and replacing the information on the whiteboard

The median time it takes to complete these activities and turn over a room (wheels out to wheels in) is 28.5 minutes.[56]

By reducing this turnover time, the delay until setup for the next surgery can start can be decreased.

Some hospitals have been able to reduce the turnover time (wheels out to wheels in) to under 22 minutes (equal to the 95th percentile)[56,57] by changing how the room turnover is performed by taking actions, such as:

- Having the entire surgical team, including the surgeon, help in turning over the room

- Using faster drying disinfectants that reduce the contact time from an average 10 minutes for bleach disinfectants to an average 5 minutes using sporicidal hydrogen peroxide/peroxyacetic acid disinfectant

- Starting to tear down the sterile instrument table and stand as soon as the last stitch has been placed

- Discontinuing mopping of the OR floor following bloodless cases

56. Data for benchmarking your OR's performance, *OR Manager* Vol. 28 No. 1 January 2012 ormanager.com/wp-content/uploads/2012/01/0112_ORM_5.Benchmark_r.pdf

57. Based on results from unpublished study of turnover times in a mid-sized community hospital.

By reducing the time needed for setup and/or cleanup, the delay between the end of one step in a process and the start of the next can be minimized as demonstrated in the example provided.

4.3.4 INCREASING CAPACITY

Sometimes shaping demand or redesigning processes are not feasible approaches for reducing or eliminating delays.

In those cases, increasing capacity may be the only way to meet demand.

Increasing capacity however does not always mean adding "more" resources.

Sometimes "increasing" capacity means nothing more than *redistributing* existing resources to more closely match demand.

Redistributing Staff

By more closely matching existing resources with demand, delays and wait times can be reduced or minimized.

The phlebotomy or blood draw process provides a good example of how resources can be redistributed to improve capacity.

After arriving at a laboratory and being checked in, patients typically have their blood drawn by a phlebotomist.

The time required by a phlebotomist to draw and label needed blood specimens in the ambulatory clinic setting has been found to average

5.5 minutes per patient.[58,59]

An outpatient laboratory staffed with 7 phlebotomists (see staff schedule below) and a daily demand of 535 patients (see distribution below) would have an average wait of 2 minutes, a maximum wait

STAFF

	8-9	9-10	10-11	11-12	12-1	1-2	2-3	3-4	4-5
A	☺	☺	☺	☺	☺		☺	☺	☺
B	☺	☺	☺	☺	☺		☺	☺	☺
C	☺	☺	☺	☺	☺		☺	☺	☺
D	☺	☺	☺	☺		☺	☺	☺	☺
E	☺	☺	☺	☺		☺	☺	☺	☺
F	☺	☺	☺	☺		☺	☺	☺	☺
G	☺	☺	☺	☺		☺	☺	☺	☺

TIME

DAILY DEMAND
Phlebotomy Blood Draw

TIME	8-9	9-10	10-11	11-12	12-1	1-2	2-3	3-4	4-5
PATIENTS	70	45	80	70	25	45	60	65	60

of 21 minutes, and 10% of patients having to wait greater than 15 minutes (see table on next page).[60]

58. Based on results of unpublished time and motion study of phlebotomist draw time in a mid-sized outpatient clinic lab.

59. Kumar et al. (2016). Time-Motion Study to Improve Sample Collection Process. *Scholars Journal of Applied Medical Sciences* (SJAMS), 2016; 4(8B):2840-2842
http://saspublisher.com/wp-content/uploads/2016/09/SJAMS-48B-2840-2842.pdf

60. Analysis based on results of discrete event simulation using Extend simulation software.

Average Wait (min)	Max Wait (min)	% Waiting	% Waiting > 15 min	Max Queue Length
2	21	23	10	11

Assuming each phlebotomist can draw 10 patients per hour (60 minutes divided by 5.5 minutes per patient), the staff needed per hour would range from 3 to 8 phlebotomists as shown below:

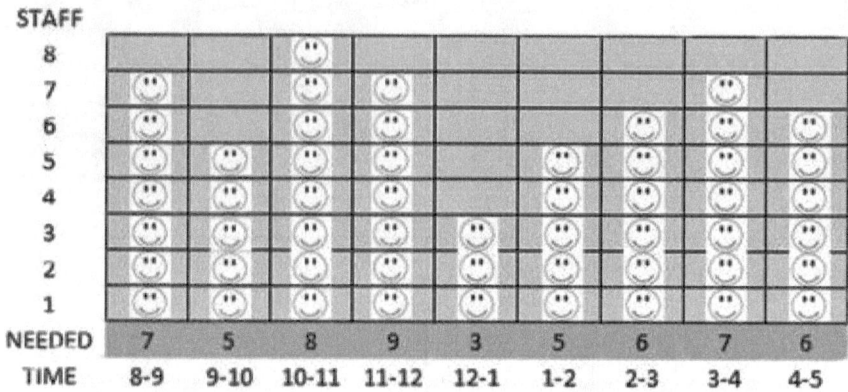

By using a combination of part-time and full-time staff and *redistributing* the 56 existing hours as shown below; the average wait time can be reduced to less than a minute, the maximum wait cut

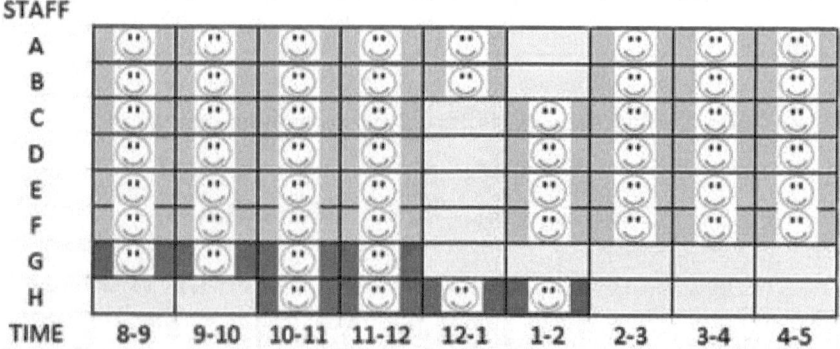

in half to 10 minutes, and none of the patients would be required to wait greater than 15 minutes (see table below).[61]

Average Wait (min)	Max Wait (min)	% Waiting	% Waiting > 15 min	Max Queue Length
1	10	6	0	8

Delays and wait times may, therefore, be able to be reduced merely by shifting existing resources to where they are needed without having to incur any additional cost.

There are times however when adding more resources is the only way to meet demand.

In these situations, labor capacity may be expanded through the use of overtime, hiring of on-call, part-time, or full-time staff, or outsourcing.

However, before additional resources are added, opportunities for cross-training of existing staff should be evaluated.

Cross-Training

Cross-training of staff effectively increases the number of employees available to perform a given task or function; without the need for hiring additional resources and their associated costs.

A good example of how cross-training can increase capacity is illustrated by looking at staffing for a typical call center.

Many multi-specialty medical groups use call centers to book patient appointments for some, if not all, of their services.

The time required to book an appointment can vary significantly from

61. Analysis based on results of discrete event simulation using Extend simulation software.

call center to call center depending on the complexity of the booking guidelines and the availability of patient appointments.

For a call center which supports three (3) different services, receives a total of 702 calls per day (with 44% of the calls for adult primary care, 33% for pediatrics, and 23% for gyn), has a total of nine (9) staff with four (4) dedicated to booking appointments for adult primary care, three (3) to booking pediatrics, and two (2) to booking gyn (see diagram below), and an average handling time per call of 4.5 minutes; patients would wait an average of 6 minutes to talk with an appointment clerk; with some patients having to wait as long as 35 minutes (see table below).[62]

Average Wait (min)	Max Wait (min)	% Waiting	% Waiting > 5 min
6	35	45	27

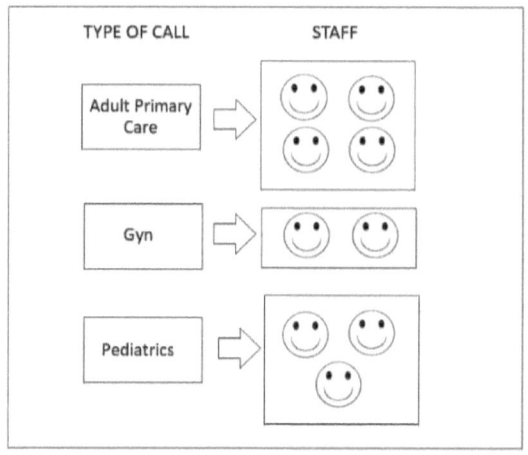

By cross-training existing staff to handle the booking of appointments for all three specialties (see diagram next page), the average time a patient would have to wait on hold to speak to an appointment clerk

62. Analysis based on results of discrete event simulation using Extend simulation software.

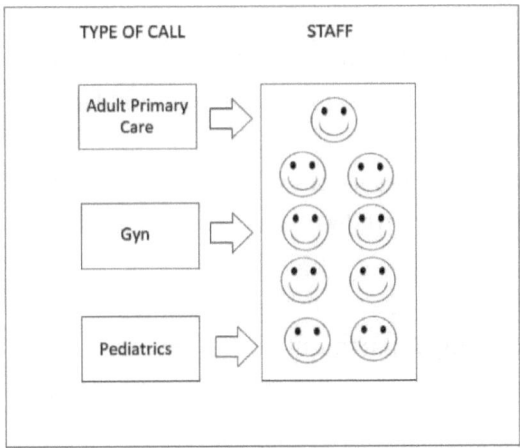

could be reduced to less than one minute; with no patient having to wait for more than 6 minutes to speak to an appointment clerk (see table below).[63]

Average Wait (min)	Max Wait (min)	% Waiting	% Waiting > 5 min
1	6	13	13

The opportunity for cross training staff should therefore always be evaluated as a way to increase capacity before additional resources are hired and additional costs incurred.

Adding Additional Resources

Sometimes, however, it's not possible to expand the capacity of existing staff or equipment; and additional resources will need to be added to reduce waiting or delays.

Adding additional resources, however, does not necessarily mean adding more full-time employees or an additional piece of equipment.

63. Analysis based on results of discrete event simulation using Extend simulation software.

Needed capacity may be added incrementally through the use of part time staff, overtime, or outsourcing rather than having to add additional fulltime staff and/or having to purchase additional equipment.

A good example of how resources can be added incrementally is the experience of a typical outpatient-based ultrasound service.

An ultrasound is a noninvasive diagnostic procedure commonly performed by imaging departments using high frequency soundwaves rather than x-rays to produce an image of targeted areas inside a patient's body.

Ultrasound is used for many reasons, including:

- Viewing the uterus and ovaries during pregnancy and monitor a developing baby's health

- Diagnosing gallbladder disease

- Evaluating blood flow

- Guiding a needle for biopsy or tumor treatment

- Examining a breast lump

- Checking a patient's thyroid gland

- Evaluating metabolic bone disease

The average length of an ultrasound appointment is 30 minutes.[64]

For a typical ultrasound service with four (4) ultrasound techs, an average appointment length of 30 minutes, and a demand of 350

64. Coombs, P. (2018). Ultrasound. *Inside Radiology*, 11/9/18
https://www.insideradiology.com.au/ultrasound/

studies per week (see distribution below), the wait time for having

WEEKLY DEMAND
Ultrasound

a procedure would average 8 days; with 52% of patients waiting over a week (see table below).[65]

Average Wait (days)	Max Wait (days)	% Waiting	% Waiting > 7 days
8	17	89	52

However, by adding a total of just one hour of overtime per day, the average patient wait can be reduced by 38% to 5 days and the percent of patients waiting more than a week reduced by 54% (see below).[65]

Average Wait (days)	Max Wait (days)	% Waiting	% Waiting > 7 days
5	12	84	24

And by adding just 2 hours of overtime per day, the average wait can be reduced by 62% while totally eliminating any patients waiting more than a week (see table next page).[65]

65. Analysis based on results of discrete event simulation using Extend simulation software for 6-month period.

Average Wait (days)	Max Wait (days)	% Waiting	% Waiting > 7 days
3	6	69	0

Although additional resources may sometimes be needed to reduce waits or delays; use of overtime, part-time staff, or outsourcing may allow additional capacity to be added incrementally to maximize results while minimizing costs.

4.3.5 IMPLEMENTING ONE-PIECE FLOW

How patients and work "flow" within and between departments affects whether patients, staff, or providers experience delays in the receipt or delivery of care or services.

When patients and work "flow", they move from one step in a process to the next without delay or interruption.

Delays and interruptions, however, are common throughout the entire healthcare delivery system because patients and work do not flow fluidly.

Instead patients and work often move slowly and laboriously through the system with frequent delays and interruptions.

Because of these problems, the Joint Commission on Accreditation of Healthcare Organizations (JCAHO) has even implemented a leadership standard called LD.04.03.11 commonly known as the "patient flow standard".

This standard states that a hospital has a process that supports the flow of patients throughout the hospital.

One of the ways that healthcare organizations can comply with this standard and minimize delays and interruptions is through the use of one-piece flow or small lot processing.

One Piece Flow [66]

One-piece flow is where an individual patient or item flows from one department or step in a process to the next without waiting or delay.

As the patient or item flows from step to step and/or department to department, whatever work is needed at that step is provided and completed before the item or patient moves to the next step of the process or treatment.

The difference between one-piece flow and the more traditional flow of work can be seen by directly comparing these two approaches relative to referrals for physical therapy.

A patient who presents to their primary care physician with lower back pain is traditionally referred to physical therapy for treatment.

In most practices this patient would have to wait several days or weeks after being referred before actually seeing the physical therapist for treatment.

Patients would also have to typically go to another facility to receive their physical therapy treatment.

In integrated health care systems that have implemented one-piece flow this patient would either be:

1. Seen in the exam room immediately following the decision by

66. More information on one-piece flow can be found in appendix X.

the doctor that the patient needed physical therapy by a physical therapist embedded in the module, or

2. Go directly to the physical therapy department in the medical office building to be seen by a physical therapist where a certain number of appointments per day have been reserved, based on historical demand, for new referral patients

By implementing one-piece flow (as illustrated above), required treatment can begin without delay; resulting in increased patient satisfaction, reduced costs, and improved outcomes. [67, 68]

Another critical element associated with one-piece flow is that the work on one patient or item is completed before proceeding to the next patient or item.

The rounding practices of hospitalists further illustrates how this principle in manufacturing called **"make one, move one"** can be applied to the delivery of healthcare.

The hospitalists in many hospitals traditionally round on all of their patients in the morning; reviewing charts, ordering some tests and services, and then spending the afternoon finishing up the work left undone at the bedside in the morning (i.e., completing notes, calling consultants, etc.).

In hospitals that have implemented the concept of one-piece flow, however, the hospitalists quickly review each patient's chart to triage and prioritize which patients need to be seen now and which patients can wait to be seen later in the day.

67. Fritz et al. (2012). Primary Care Referral of Patients with low back pain to Physical Therapy: impact on future healthcare utilization and costs. *Spine* (Phila Pa 1976). 2012 Dec 1;37(25):2114-21.
https://www.ncbi.nlm.nih.gov/pubmed/22614792/

68. Strauss, A. (2018). Physical Therapy + Primary Care = Improved Access for Veterans, *MED Magazine*, Aug 28, 2018
https://www.midwestmedicaledition.com/2018/08/28/179217/physical-therapy-primary-care-improved-access-for-veterans

As the hospitalists see each patient, they spend as long as is needed talking to nurses, calling consultants, and entering and completing all notes, orders, documentation, and billing; rather than deferring some of these activities to a later time.

Only when they have finished all these activities do they move on to the next patient.

At one hospital where this concept was applied, the hospitalists reported significant improvements to their workflow; leading to reductions in their workday of close to 90 minutes each.[69]

Batching of work is another common practice in the delivery of healthcare.

It is a widely held belief that batching or aggregating work and then completing it all at once is more efficient than completing one entire task before moving on to the next task.

In many cases, however, the opposite is true and batching of work actually creates inefficiency and unnecessary delay.

A good example is how physicians in clinic often handle the messages they receive from their patients.

In many clinic practices, the doctors hold on to or "batch" their messages until the end of the day.

They then return all the messages they received throughout the day at that time.

Rather than "batching" messages and calling patients at the end of the day, physicians in practices that have adopted one-piece flow respond

69. Mazanec, D. (2016). The Toyota Model in Healthcare Delivery: One Piece Flow. *1776*, February 26, 2016, https://www.1776.vc/insights/toyota-model-healthcare-delivery/

to messages as they are received, between patients, or during the time freed up when patients no show.

By not "batching" and holding messages till the end of the day, patients receive a timelier response from their physician while eliminating a bolus of work for the doctor at the end of the day.

In addition, repeat calls from patients and unnecessary visits to the ED or Urgent Care may also be avoided.

Small-Lot Processing

Another example of "batching" in healthcare is how blood is drawn on hospitalized patients.

Blood is drawn on most hospitalized patients first thing in the morning so that the results are available to physicians when making their morning rounds.

In most hospitals, the phlebotomists draw the blood from all the patients on a unit before tubing or taking the specimens down to the laboratory for processing.

This "batching" of specimens results in both delays and "*mura*" or "unevenness" in how specimens are received by the lab.

While implementing one-piece flow and sending each sample to the lab after being drawn is neither practical nor efficient, a hybrid approach can be used known as "small-lot processing".

Rather than drawing a specimen and then immediately sending it down to the lab as would be done with one-piece flow; with small-lot processing, several specimens are collected and then tubed or taken down to the lab for processing.

This reduces the overall turnaround time; enabling results to be made available to the unit faster than if specimens wait to be batched before being sent to the lab for processing (see below).

BATCH PROCESSING   **SMALL LOT PROCESSING**

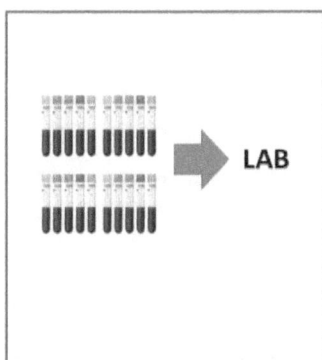
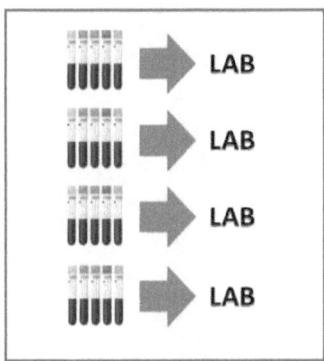

For a typical twenty (20) bed hospital unit, the lab results for <u>all</u> patients would be available 8% sooner (177 minutes versus 193 minutes) if specimens were collected and sent to the lab in small lots rather than batched.[70]

In addition, the average turnaround time would be 60% shorter (43 minutes vs 111 minutes).[70]

Small-lot processing therefore creates a balance between improved efficiency and improved turnaround time for those situations where one-piece flow can-not be effectively implemented.

70. Analysis based on results of discrete event simulation using Extend simulation software assuming the specimens collected from the unit are tubed down to the lab in small lots (i.e., once specimens were collected from 5 patients) instead of being held until all 20 specimens have been collected, each specimen takes seven (7) minutes to collect, the time to prepare and tube samples is 5 minutes, and processing time in the lab is thirty (30) minutes per 10 specimens.

4.4   "Treating" INVENTORY waste

Inventory is typically defined as the supply of materials on hand or needed to manufacture a product.

But what about in healthcare where the product is the delivery of care to a patient?

Delivery of this "product" requires more than just materials and supplies.

The delivery of care requires materials and supplies like medications, syringes, and sutures.

But the delivery of care also requires a supply or "inventory" of patient beds, patient appointments, and diagnostic and therapeutic equipment.

Waste of these resources can occur in numerous ways depending on what type of "inventory" is involved; ranging from the expiration of medications, unfilled or unkept appointments, to needed beds waiting to be cleaned for a patient admitted from the Emergency Room.

Reducing or eliminating this type of "*MUDA*" or "waste" can require actions that involve changes in inventory management practices, physician practices, scheduling practices, and utilization practices.

Some of the most common actions that can be taken to reduce or eliminate these different types of "inventory" waste include:

- Standardizing practices

- Pooling

- Simplifying processes

- Implementing Just in Time (JIT) practices

- Setting up Kanban systems

4.4.1 STANDARDIZING PRACTICES

Physicians have been culturized from early in their careers to function autonomously in their practice of medicine.

As a result of this culture of autonomy in thinking and decision-making, there is tremendous variation in individual physician practice.

This variation in practice can lead to waste in supplies, appointments, and bed "inventories".

By standardizing practice and reducing the amount of variation between physicians, unnecessary and costly waste can be reduced or eliminated.

A good example of how greater standardization can reduce inventory "waste" is the stocking of electrothermal bipolar vessel sealing devices (EBVS) in the operating room.

An electrothermal bipolar vessel sealing device (EBVS) is an instrument used for cauterizing arteries and blood vessels during both open and minimally invasive surgery.

There are a number of manufacturers of vessel sealing devices; each with slightly different features, design, and cost (often several hundred dollars difference).

Different surgeons often prefer one device over another, resulting in operating rooms maintaining an inventory of several different brands of vessel sealers; increasing both the amount and cost of inventory maintained.

By getting surgeons to agree to standardize and use just one brand of vessel sealer, the amount and cost of inventory maintained by the operating room can be reduced by tens of thousands of dollars per year.

At one hospital, standardization of supplies in the operating room resulted in an average 20% reduction in supply cost per case, with no significant change in operative time, total time in OR, or length of stay.[71]

Even greater reductions in the amount and costs of inventory can be achieved if all supplies and instruments used throughout the hospital can be standardized.[72]

Besides impacting supply and instrument inventories, differences in individual physician practice can also impact the inventory of appointments of individual physicians or services.

Studies have shown that there is significant variation in return visit intervals and referral practices between primary care physicians.

These differences, which can impact appointment utilization and access, often have little correlation with a patient's actual medical condition.

According to one study, the patient's medical condition accounted for

71. Avansino et al. (2013). Standardization of operative equipment reduces cost. *J Pediatr Surg*. 2013 Sep; 48(9):1843-9. doi: 10.1016/j.jpedsurg.2012.11.045
https://www.ncbi.nlm.nih.gov/pubmed/24074655

72. Annual Supply Chain Savings Opportunity Reaches $25.7 Billion for U.S. Hospitals, Navigant Analysis Finds, *Navigant*, Nov 13, 2019
https://www.navigant.com/news/corporate-news/2019/supply-chain-analysis-2019

only 18% of the observed variation in return visit intervals.[73]

The remaining variation was attributable primarily to physician preference and practice.[73]

These findings were further reinforced by another study which looked at return visit intervals for patients with chronic, stable, uncomplicated hypertension.

This study found that 37.3% of the physicians surveyed brought these patients back in less than 6 months despite compelling evidence in the literature that return visit intervals of 6 months to 1 year were appropriate for patients in this condition.[74]

Such variation in return visit practices can adversely impact appointment inventories and reduce patient access for appointments.

A good example of how variation in return visit intervals can impact appointment inventories and access is documented in a study of physician management practices of patients with diabetes, hypertension, and hyperlipidemia.

According to this study, 69% of patients with diabetes, hypertension, or hyperlipidemia were scheduled for return visits in less than 6 months.[75]

After working with the physicians to standardize and extend return intervals, the percentage of patients that were scheduled for return visits in less than 6 months had fallen to 38%; reducing provider visits by

73. Schwartz et al. (1999). Setting the Revisit Interval in Primary Care. *J Gen Intern Med*. 1999 Apr; 14(4): 230–235
https://www.ncbi.nlm.nih.gov/pmc/articles/PMC1496560/

74. Pol, E. (2016). Physician Empanelment and Patient Re-Visit Intervals in the Era of Healthcare Reform: An Analysis of Appropriate Follow-up Times for Patients with Chronic Conditions in a Federally Qualified Health Center (FQHC),
https://nmfonline.org/wp-content/uploads/2016/02/Escobedo-Pol-Evelyn-Paper.pdf

27% without any adverse impact on glycemic control or other outcome measures.[75]

Similar findings were found for physician referral practices.

More than a third of patients are referred to a specialist each year; with specialist visits constituting more than half of all outpatient visits.[76]

The decision as to when to make a referral has been found to vary widely, with some primary care providers making more than five times as many referrals per patient or per visit as other providers.[76]

Several studies found that less than 40% of the observed variation in provider referral practices can be explained by patient characteristics or medical condition.[77]

The remaining variation was attributable primarily to physician preference and practice.[77]

A number of studies have also shown that between 16% to 30% of all referrals are unnecessary or inappropriate;[76] reducing the inventory of appointments available for patients that really require access.

The use of referral guidelines is one way to combat inappropriate referrals and the "wasting" of available appointments.

75. Schectman et al. (2005). Prolonging the Return Visit Interval in Primary Care. *American Journal of Medicine*, Vol 118 #4 April 2005
https://sites.ualberta.ca/~dcl3/ABCDreview/papers/2005_Schectman_10876.pdf

76. Mehrotra et al. (2011). Dropping the Baton: Specialty Referrals in the United States. *Milbank Q*. 2011 Mar; 89(1): 39–68.doi: 10.1111/j.1468-0009.2011.00619.x
https://www.ncbi.nlm.nih.gov/pmc/articles/PMC3160594/

77. O'Donnell, C. (2000). Variation in GP referral rates: what can we learn from the literature? *Fam Pract*. 2000 Dec;17(6):462-71.
https://www.ncbi.nlm.nih.gov/pubmed/11120716

Referral guidelines can assist primary care physicians make appropriate referral decisions by not only providing criteria as to when a referral is indicated, but by also providing direction as to how to workup and manage the patient prior to referral (see example below for tinnitus).

REFERRAL GUIDELINES FOR TINNITUS			
Diagnosis/Symptoms	Evaluation	Management Options	Referral Guideline
Chronic Bilateral	Any associated symptoms? Cerumen?	Clear cerumen and check TM. If TM clear, no treatment	No referral indicated unless tinnitus is disabling or associated with hearing loss, aural discharge or vertigo – category 4
Unilateral or recent onset	Any associated symptoms? Cerumen?	Clear cerumen and check TM. If symptoms persist, refer	Referral indicated, especially if it is disabling or associated with hearing loss, aural discharge or vertigo – category 4
Pulsatile	TM normal or (vascular) mass behind drum Auscultate carotid vessels	Referral	Referral is indicated in all cases. If there is a middle ear mass, there is a strong possibility of a glomus tumor

A number of studies have shown that the use of referral guidelines can cut the number of inappropriate referrals in half [79, 80], while significantly improving the quality of workup performed by the primary care provider prior to referral of the patient to the specialist.[81]

A better workup of patients prior to referral and a reduction in the number and rate of inappropriate referrals was found to result in improved utilization of available appointment "inventory", reducing

79. Mahalingam et al. Reducing inappropriate referrals to secondary care: our experiences with the ENT Emergency clinic, Quality in Primary Care.
http://primarycare.imedpub.com/reducing-inappropriate-referrals-to-secondary-care-our-experiences-with-the-ent-emergency-clinic.php?aid=10

80. Daultrey et al. (2014). Improving Appropriateness of Referral to ENT Emergency Clinic: A Completed Audit Loop. *The Otorhinolaryngologist* 7(1) :40-43 · January 2014
https://www.researchgate.net/publication/289751823_Improving_appropriateness_of_referral_to_ENT_emergency_clinic_A_completed_audit_loop

81. Clarke et al. (2009). The REFER Project: Realistic Effective Facilitation of Elective Referral for Elective Surgical Referral. *NCCSDO*, October 2009

wait times and improving patient access to care.[82]

4.4.2 POOLING RESOURCES

Pooling is the combining, consolidating, and sharing of resources such as inventory to optimize service, access, efficiency, or performance.

A good example of how pooling can optimize "inventory" is the use of operating rooms.

The operating room is one of the most expensive areas of the hospital and it is important that the available "inventory" of surgical blocks or time not be wasted.

Many hospitals have designated one of the operating rooms in their hospital strictly for emergency surgeries, with the belief that this practice will expedite emergency access to an operating room.

Several studies have shown that dedicating an operating room for emergency surgeries in fact reduces access to the operating room, increasing wait times to get a patient to required surgery.[83]

Pooling of all available block time and performing both scheduled and emergency surgeries in the same operating rooms, on the other hand, has been found to decrease the time emergency cases have to wait to get access to a room.

One study showed that pooled use of operating rooms resulted in reduction of the average waiting time for emergency surgery from 74 minutes to 8 minutes.[83]

82. Clarke et al. (2009). Can guidelines improve referral to elective surgical specialties for adults? A systematic review. *Quality Safety Health Care* (2009).
https://qualitysafety.bmj.com/content/qhc/early/2010/03/04/qshc.2008.029918.full.pdf

83. Kolker, A. (2012). By Management Engineering for Effective Healthcare Delivery: Principles and Applications IGI Global, 2012

This finding was corroborated by another study using simulation which found that emergency cases had to wait twice as long to get access to an operating room when facilities utilized dedicated operating rooms versus pooled operating rooms.[83]

Besides having an adverse impact on wait times, dedicating an operating room strictly for emergency surgeries was also found to be less efficient than squeezing emergency surgeries into pooled operating rooms.

While the median utilization of operating rooms nationally averaged 75% (and 93% at the 90th percentile),[84] the utilization of dedicated operating rooms averaged only 39%;[83] demonstrating how the practice of pooling can improve both the efficiency and utilization of available resources.

4.4.3 SIMPLIFYING PROCESSES

Processes are often dynamic; evolving over time with band aids and workarounds incorporated into the workflow to address problems, stakeholder complaints/concerns, or changes in technology.

Rather than making the workflow simpler and more efficient, these band aids and workarounds often add increased complexity and inefficiency to the process.

Such complexity can result in loss, shrinkage, or waste of "inventory".

A good example of how simplifying a process can cut inventory "waste" in healthcare is patient no-shows for appointments.

83. Kolker, A. (2012). By Management Engineering for Effective Healthcare Delivery: Principles and Applications, IGI Global, 2012

84. Foster, T. (2012). Data for benchmarking your OR's performance. *OR Manager*, Vol 28 No 1 Jan 2012
https://www.ormanager.com/wp-content/uploads/2012/01/0112_ORM_5.Benchmark_r.pdf

Besides "wasting" physician and staff time, patient no-shows reduce the availability of appointments for other patients; resulting in delays in their treatment or their use of other more expensive forms of care (i.e., urgent care or ER).

Patient no-shows remain a common problem for physicians.

According to one survey, forty-four (44) percent of physicians surveyed stated that their biggest challenge was patient no-shows.[85]

While the rate of patient no-shows varies from physician to physician and specialty to specialty, patient no-show rates average 19% nationally.[86]

One of the major reasons for patient no-shows is excessive delays between patients' requests to be seen and patients actually seeing the physician.[87, 88]

Physicians have historically used a number of different appointment types with different durations and different uses for scheduling patients (with some physicians or services having up to 20 to 30 different appointment types).

While intended to better balance physician time with patient clinical needs, the use of multiple appointment types can restrict how

85. Harrop, C. (2017). Practice leaders report their biggest challenges with appointments are no-shows and appointment availability. *MGMA STAT*, October 3, 2017 https://www.mgma.com/data/data-stories/practice-leaders-report-their-biggest-challenges-w

86. Gebhart, T. (2017). No-Show Management in Primary Care: A Quality Improvement Project. Scholar Archive, April 13, 2017 https://pdfs.semanticscholar.org/09a1/a915c0b60729dc66bb6fb08aedeb5e74e304.pdf

87. Anisi et al. (2018). Appointments: Factors Contributing to Patient No-Show in Outpatient Hospital Missed Clinics in Tehran, Iran. *Shiraz E-Medical Journal*, July 2, 2018 http://emedicalj.com/en/articles/63238.html

88. Maximizing Patient Access and Scheduling : An MGMA Research and Analysis Report August 2017, https://www.mgma.com/MGMA/media/files/data/MGMAR-A_PatientAccess_Excerpt.pdf

appointments are utilized; leading to increased patient wait times for appointments.

A number of studies have found that the length of time patients must wait for an appointment can be reduced by simplifying or reducing the number of different appointment types.[89, 90]

Several healthcare organizations which have "simplified" their appointment types and appointment booking guidelines have successfully cut their no-show rates in half; [91, 92] demonstrating how simplification of complex processes can help reduce unnecessary "waste" of limited inventory.

4.4.4   JUST IN TIME

The concept of Just in Time or JIT is that products or services that are required are provided "just in time" to the customer.

In other words, **what** the customer wants, **how** the customer wants it, and **when** the customer wants or needs it.

Although the principles of JIT are most commonly associated with the management of materials and supplies, they also have applicability to many other areas of healthcare including management of appointments and space.

89. Giachetti, R. (2008). A Simulation Study of Interventions to Reduce Appointment Lead-Time and Patient No-Show Rate. *Proceedings of the 2008 Winter Simulation Conference*
https://www.informs-sim.org/wsc08papers/178.pdf

90. Reduce scheduling complexity, Institute for Healthcare Improvement
http://www.ihi.org/resources/Pages/Changes/ReduceSchedulingComplexity.aspx

91. Lynn et al. (2016). Open access scheduling: Improving access to rural healthcare. *Journal of Nursing Education and Practice*, Vol 6 No 9, 2016
http://www.sciedu.ca/journal/index.php/jnep/article/viewFile/8751/5762

92. Improving Access and Efficiency in Primary Care at HealthServe Community Health Center, HealthServe Community Health Center (a Moses Cone clinic) Greensboro, North Carolina, USA, IHI Improvement Stories
http://www.ihi.org/resources/Pages/ImprovementStories/ImprovingAccessandEfficiencyinPrimaryCareatHealthServe.aspx

Materials and Supplies

Healthcare depends on the availability of materials and supplies like medications, syringes, and sutures.

A significant amount of these supplies, however, end up being "wasted" when items pass their expiration dates, similar products are stocked from different manufacturers to meet physician preferences, new and updated products become available, and inventory management practices are inadequate or absent.

A good example of how Just in Time (JIT) principles can be used to reduce the waste of supply inventory is the management of disposable supplies in the operating room.

A large number of disposable supplies are used in the operating room.

To minimize delays during surgery, scrub techs often open all of the disposable supplies required prior to the start of surgery.

The result is that a number of disposables, some of which are quite costly, go unused and end up having to be disposed of or "wasted".

Studies have found that on average 13% of the total nonpayroll cost of a case ends up being wasted due to disposable supplies being opened but unused.[93]

With a "just in time" approach, the scrub tech would open any disposables **just** before the item is needed by the surgeon, rather than prior to the start of surgery; reducing "waste" and the need to dispose of costly opened, but unused sterile supplies.

93. Zygourakis et al. (2017). Operating room waste: disposable supply utilization in neurosurgical procedures. *J Neurosurg*. 2017 Feb;126(2):620-625. doi: 10.3171/2016.2.JNS152442. Epub 2016 May 6
https://www.ncbi.nlm.nih.gov/pubmed/27153160

The principles of Just in Time (JIT) are not limited to just the OR, but can be applied to the management of materials and supplies throughout an entire facility or organization; allowing for the recapture of even more costs and greater savings.

Appointments

Patient access to physicians and associated medical care is often limited by the number of available <u>unbooked</u> appointments a physician has.

The lack of a sufficient inventory of appointments available for booking can lead to long patient waits to see a doctor.

A good example of how JIT can reduce the "waste" of appointment "inventory" is the open access model of patient scheduling.

Traditionally physicians' schedules are booked, sometimes weeks in advance, with routine, return, or follow-up visits.

Patients with urgent problems would typically be offered any available appointment or "possibly" squeezed into the schedule.

This scheduling practice often results in clogged physician schedules, long waits for routine appointments, and highly dissatisfied patients <u>and</u> physicians.

The open access appointment model is built on the principle of leaving the majority of appointments "open" and providing a patient with an appointment the same day they call...or "just in time".

This change in scheduling practice has resulted in improved utilization of appointments, improved patient access, and improved physician and patient satisfaction.

A study of six (6) primary care clinics found that the mean wait time till the third available appointment, a common measure of access by many medical groups, decreased by 60% following implementation of open access in their clinics.[94]

Another study found that physician practices that had implemented open access were seeing 75% of their patients within 2 days versus only 57% for practices that had booked their patients using traditional scheduling models.[95]

Patient satisfaction with wait times was also 5 percentage points higher for clinics that had implemented open access compared to practices still booking patients using traditional scheduling models.[95]

By freeing up the "inventory" of appointments for patients needing to be seen during regular clinic hours, open access scheduling also reduced the utilization of urgent care or emergency room services by those patients who had previously been unable to get appointments in a timely manner.[96]

As with other forms of inventory, use of a "just in time" approach can prevent inefficient utilization or "waste" of resources (appointments, procedure slots, or other needed services); translating into reduced wait times and improved patient or customer satisfaction.

Space

The availability of adequate space to meet demand is a challenge in

94. Mehrotra et al. (2008). Implementation of Open Access Scheduling in Primary Care: A Cautionary Tale. *Ann Int Med* 2008 Jun 17; 148(12):915-922 https://www.ncbi.nlm.nih.gov/pmc/articles/PMC2587225/

95. Salisbury et al. (2007). Does Advanced Access improve access to primary health care? Questionnaire survey of patients. *Br J Gen Pract.* 2007 Aug 1; 57(541): 615–621 https://www.ncbi.nlm.nih.gov/pmc/articles/PMC2099666/

96. O' Hare, C. & Corlett, J. (2004). The Outcomes of Open Access Scheduling. *Fam Pract Manag.* 2004 Feb;11(2):35-38., https://www.aafp.org/fpm/2004/0200/p35.html

most hospitals and medical facilities.

Demand for hospital beds, treatment areas, and operating rooms often exceeds the available "inventory" of these limited "space" resources; resulting in long patient waits or backlogs.

A good example of how JIT can be used to help reduce "wasting" of any of these available spaces is the Emergency Room.

Emergency Rooms are notorious for long patient waits.

One of the factors contributing to these excessive waits is the lack of available treatment rooms.

Treatment rooms often get tied up with patients that emergency room physicians have not yet diagnosed and/or treated when required test results have not been received back from the lab or diagnostic imaging.

Labs are typically ordered on 56%–76% of the patients that present to the Emergency Room.[97, 98]

Lab specimens are typically collected and sent or transported to a central laboratory where the specimens are processed and analyzed.

Turnaround time from collection of these lab specimens till reporting of results can typically take from 30 minutes to over an hour depending on

97. Ngo et al. (2017). Frequency that Laboratory Tests Influence Medical Decisions. *The Journal of Applied Laboratory Medicine* January 2017 pg 410-414. https://doi.org/10.1373/jalm.2016.021634 http://jalm.aaccjnls.org/content/1/4/410

98. Lewandrowski, K. (2011). POC testing in the emergency department: Strategies to improve clinical and operational outcomes. acutecaretesting.org, October 2011, https://acutecaretesting.org/en/articles/poc-testing-in-the-emergency-department-strategies-to-improve-clinical-and-operational-outcomes

the type of test, the institution, and the time of day.[99]

During this time, the room is tied up and unavailable for use for diagnosis or treatment of other patients.

Turnaround times for lab results, however, can be reduced significantly by using moderate or complex point of care testing.

Use of moderate or complex point of care testing, which can be performed "just in time" in the emergency room using handheld or portable devices, can eliminate the need to send specimens to the lab; freeing up treatment rooms sooner and allowing faster room turnover to accommodate another patient.

One study found that the turnaround time for test results was reduced from an average of 83 minutes to an average of 15 minutes following the transition to point of care testing.[100]

Another study found that the length of stay in the Emergency Room was reduced by an average 1.9 hours or 27% in those hospitals where point of care testing was introduced.[100]

By providing test results "just in time", point of care testing allows emergency room physicians to diagnose, treat, and discharge or admit their patients faster; freeing up treatment room "inventory" to accommodate other patients.

99. Li et al. (2015). The Effect of Laboratory Testing on Emergency Department Length of Stay: A Multihospital Longitudinal Study Applying a Cross-classified Random-effect Modeling Approach. *Academic Emergency Medicine*, Jan 6, 2015, https://onlinelibrary.wiley.com/doi/full/10.1111/acem.12565

100. Singer et al. (2005). Point-of-Care Testing Reduces Length of Stay in Emergency Department Chest Pain Patients. *Annals of Emergency Medicine*, June 2005 Volume 45, Issue 6, Pages 587–591 https://www.annemergmed.com/article/S0196-0644(04)01712-3/abstract?code=ymem-site

4.4.5 *KANBAN*

Kanban is a Japanese term meaning "signboard" or "signal".

This term is commonly used to refer to an inventory management system which signals the need to replenish supplies or materials.

Unlike in manufacturing, *"kanban"* may assume a number of different forms to accommodate the many different types of inventory managed in healthcare (i.e., supplies, exam rooms, hospital beds, etc.).

Bin or Card Systems

One of the most common types of *"kanban"* systems is the "two-bin" system which is used in many pharmacies.

> *Note: A reorder card placed in a single bin may also be used in lieu of a second bin to signal the need for replenishment.*

This system utilizes two bins of supplies; one which contains working stock and the other which contains reserve stock.

When the bin containing the working stock is depleted, it is replaced with the bin which contains the reserve stock (see illustration on next page).

The empty bin serves as the "signal" that the supplies or materials contained in the working bin need to be replenished or reordered (see appendix X for how to calculate reserve bin quantity).

"Kanban" systems have been implemented in many healthcare organizations.

Many of these organizations have reported declines in the number of stockouts experienced, the amount of inventory needed, and declines in the per patient cost of care following conversion to a "kanban" system for management of their supply inventory.

One hospital realized a 13% reduction in inventory levels, along with the recovery of 24% of floor space, following their conversion to a "kanban" system.[101]

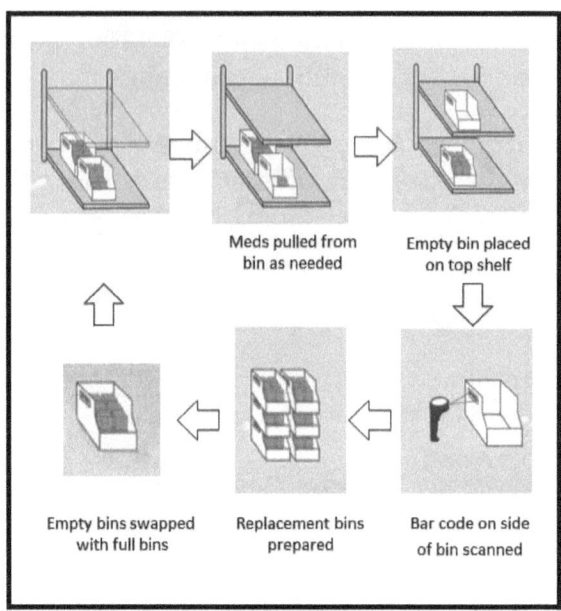

Meds pulled from bin as needed

Empty bin placed on top shelf

Empty bins swapped with full bins

Replacement bins prepared

Bar code on side of bin scanned

Another hospital realized an 85% reduction in its incidence of stockouts following conversion to a *kanban* system, while a third realized per patient cost of care reductions of 3.7%.[101, 102]

These results illustrate why *"kanban"* systems are often found to be more effective than par level or min-max systems for managing the inventory of supplies in many healthcare organizations.

101. Carter, A. (2016). Two-Bin Kanban: Ordering Impact at Navy Medical Center San Diego. Acquisition Research Program Sponsored Report Series, June 17, 2016
https://apps.dtic.mil/dtic/tr/fulltext/u2/1016680.pdf

102. Spear, S. (2005). Fixing Healthcare from the Inside, Today. *Harvard Business Review*, September 2005
https://hbr.org/2005/09/fixing-health-care-from-the-inside-today

Lights

Another *"kanban"* commonly found in healthcare to signal or trigger that action is needed is the exam room light frequently placed outside a physician's exam room.

The exam room light serves as a signal or visual cue to the nurse or physician that some action is required.

The exam room light can be used to signal to the nurse that a room is vacant and ready for the next patient, that the patient in the room is ready for discharge, or that the room is ready to be cleaned.

The exam room light can also be used to signal to the physician that a patient has been roomed, prepped, and is ready to be seen by the physician.

Using such a *"kanban"* facilitates quicker turnover and use of the available "inventory" of exam rooms; eliminating delays and allowing work to flow more efficiently in the clinic.

Kanban Boards

Bed management boards are another form of *"kanban"*.

These boards use color-coded icons to visually signal staff of pending discharges, pending admissions, unoccupied beds, etc. (see example on next page).

Based on the color of a given icon, staff know what actions need to be taken (i.e., clean a bed), when they need to be taken (i.e., now), and where they need to be taken (i.e., unit 1 bed 4); helping reduce delays in communication and improving the turnover of available beds.

These reductions in bed turnover time can translate into improved patient flow, increased throughput, increased revenue, and improved patient and physician satisfaction.

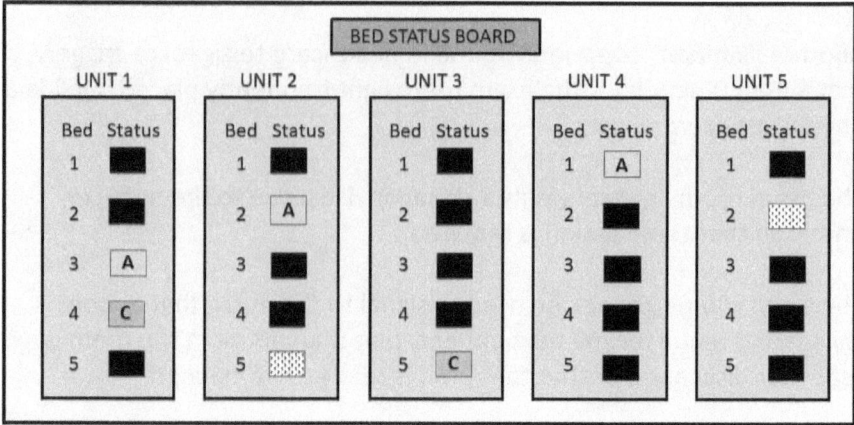

At one hospital that implemented a *"kanban"* board for bed management, the hospital experienced a 53% decrease in bed turnaround time and an 85% decrease in admission turnaround time.[104]

As a result of turning around their beds faster, the hospital realized $1.7 million in savings from decreased costs and increased revenue.[104]

Whether used for supply management, staff management, or bed management, the use of *"kanban"* allows limited resources to be utilized more effectively and efficiently; saving time, energy, and money.

4.5   "Treating" HUMAN TALENT waste

It takes more than just processes to get things done.

It also takes people.

Healthcare is very labor intensive and human talent represents one of

104. Using Tracking Tools to Improve Patient Flow in Hospitals, California Healthcare Foundation Issue Brief August 2011
https://www.chcf.org/wp-content/uploads/2017/12/PDF-UsingPatientTrackingToolsInHospitals.pdf

the greatest expenses for most healthcare organizations.

Unutilized, underutilized, or inefficiently utilized staff can therefore be a costly "waste".

So, what actions can be taken to reduce or eliminate the waste of human talent available in your organization?

Common actions that can be taken include:

- Simplifying or eliminating non value-added work

- Staffing to TAKT time (move staff/move work)

- Reducing defects

- Improving flow and load leveling

- Dealing with poor performers

4.5.1   WORK SIMPLIFICATION

Processes consist of a number of steps or tasks.

Often these processes are more complex than they need to be and may be simplified by taking one or more of the following actions:

- Eliminating or consolidating steps

- Redesigning tasks or workflow

- Automating steps or using new technologies

Eliminating or Consolidating Steps

Sometimes one or more of the steps in a process are redundant, are no longer necessary, or add no value...and can be eliminated or consolidated.

A simple example is the pulling of supplies for surgery.

Many surgeries require a significant number of disposable supplies ranging from sponges to blades and sutures.

All the supplies required for an upcoming case are typically pulled by either a nurse or a supply tech from the storeroom according to a pick list and then placed on a case cart that is wheeled into the operating room before the start of each case.

These supplies are then unloaded from the cart and set up in the operating room in preparation for the surgery.

Picking the supplies for these cases is a very labor-intensive process.

This step can be eliminated for a number of surgeries by purchasing custom packs from a vendor which contain most, if not all, of the disposable supplies required.

Besides eliminating or reducing the time required for nurses or techs to pull supplies, the use of surgical packs also reduces the time required to unload, unwrap, and set up the supplies.

One hospital that converted to use of surgical packs in their operating room reduced the time its nurses spent pulling, unwrapping, and setting up supplies for its ortho cases by approximately forty (40) percent.[105]

105. Trygged, I. & Krusell, O. (2016). Reduction of Changeover Times Between Surgeries, Master's Thesis in Quality and Operations Management, Chalmers University of Technology, 2016
http://publications.lib.chalmers.se/records/fulltext/241301/241301.pdf

Other hospitals showed that the use of procedure packs reduced the resources required for the daily pre-selection of surgical products by more than 30%, the resources required for picking of items for individual surgical procedures by 57%, and operating room set-up times by more than 36%; freeing up nurses and scrub techs to focus on other key patient care activities.[106]

By eliminating or consolidating any unnecessary or redundant steps in a process, workflows can be streamlined and the "waste" of human talent reduced; resulting in increased staff and/or physician efficiency and productivity.

Redesigning Tasks or Workflow

Another way that processes can be simplified to reduce the "waste" of human talent is by **redesigning** or **reorganizing** the way a task is performed.

A good example of how a process or task can be redesigned is the approach used by one hospital to simplify their process when performing cataract surgeries.

Prior to the redesign, the average wait time for cataract surgery was 46 days with an average of four cataract surgeries being performed per block or half day.

By applying the principles of work simplification and making the following changes to their process to remove "waste" from the process (see table on next page), the number of surgeries that could be performed were increased to 11 cases per block, nearly tripling staff

106. Improvement of Operating Theatre Capacity by the Use of procedure packs, Klinik-Management-Consulting, Germany (2002)
www.Rocialle.com/cpt/

and physician productivity.[107]

BEFORE	AFTER	PRINCIPLE
Use Retrobulbar block	Use topical anesthetic *Rationale: reduces time needed to apply and take effect; safer*	Reduce setup time
No criteria used to determine order in which patients scheduled	Right eyed surgeries scheduled followed by left eyed surgeries *Rationale: minimizes need to reposition microscope*	Reduce setup time Eliminate redundant steps
Patient undresses fully	Patient undresses from waist up *Rationale: reduces time for patient to change*	Eliminate unnecessary steps
Full documentation	Short form documentation *Rationale: reduces documentation time*	Eliminate non-value added steps
Surgical table used	Eye gurney used *Rationale: Eliminates need to transfer patient to surgical table*	Eliminate unnecessary step
Re-sterilized trays from earlier surgeries for later surgeries	Had enough trays for each scheduled surgery *Rationale: Eliminates delays from waiting for re-sterilized trays to be returned*	Minimize handoffs

This increase in productivity was achieved without an increase in the vitrectomy rate or any other measures of surgical quality.

> *Note: A vitrectomy is a procedure performed to address a complication often associated with cataract surgery.*

107. Based on results from unpublished study of impact of process changes on cataract surgery in a mid-sized community hospital.

With the increased volume of cases that could be performed per block, the average wait time for cataract surgery dropped by over 80% to below 2 weeks; resulting in improved patient and physician satisfaction.

By redesigning and/or reorganizing the way work is performed, processes and workflows can be made more efficient; helping to improve productivity and reduce the "waste" of human talent.

Automation or Use of Technology

Technology can also help reduce the "waste" of human talent by simplifying the way work is being done.

A good example of how work can be simplified through the use of technology is by looking at how clinicians in mental health document their notes.

In many practices, session notes are still being hand written or typed into an electronic medical record (EMR) by the clinician.

The speed at which these notes can be entered into the medical record can vary from about 20 words per minute for a clinician who uses the hunt and peck method to about 40 words per minute for a clinician with proficient typing skills.[108]

While a typical clinician may be able to type at a rate of 30 - 40 words per minute, they can typically speak at a rate of at least 150 words per minute.[109]

By using speech recognition transcription software, the amount of time

108. Williams, S. (2015). Can Dragon Speech Recognition beat the world touch typing record? IT ProPortal, Mar 10, 2015 https://www.itproportal.com/2015/03/10/can-dragon-speech-recognition-beat-world-touch-typing-record/

109. What is the average dictation speed, Reference.com, https://www.reference.com/business-finance/average-dictation-speed-c4496ed481457f6c

that clinicians must spend on documentation can be significantly reduced.

A study at one mental health facility showed that the amount of time clinicians spent entering notes was reduced 50% following installation of such software, without any significant increase in errors.[110]

A study at another mental health facility showed a decrease in average typing time by clinicians of 51 minutes which was accompanied by a corresponding increase in clinical contact time with patients.[111]

In addition, the average turnaround time for letters and reports dropped from 6 -7 days to just 1 -2 days following implementation of the voice recognition technology.[110]

Use of automation and technology, however, does not always end up streamlining processes and reducing inefficiency and the "waste" of human talent.

Studies have shown that at least 40% of new technology projects fail, are abandoned, or do not end up meeting their intended goal or purpose.[111]

A good example of how new technology in healthcare can fail to meet its intended goal is provided by one organization's efforts to implement appointment self-registration kiosks at its clinics.

The leadership of this organization felt that labor costs could be reduced and service improved (i.e. reduced patient lines) by use of technology which could streamline the patient check-in and registration process for patient appointments.

110. Amirault, B. (2013). Mental health professionals benefit from voice recognition programs. Barton Associates, July 19, 2013
https://www.bartonassociates.com/blog/mental-health-professionals-benefit-from-voice-recognition-programs/?p=2013/07/19/mental-health-professionals-benefit-from-voice-recognition-programs/

111. Kaplan B. & Harris-Salamone, K. (2009). Health IT Success and Failure: Recommendations from Literature and an AMIA workshop. *J Am Med Inform Assoc.* 2009 May-Jun; 16(3): 291–299
https://www.ncbi.nlm.nih.gov/pmc/articles/PMC2732244/

Custom built kiosks were set up in the lobbies of several high-volume clinics for patients to use for self-registration and check-in.

Although the availability and convenience of the kiosks were vigorously promoted to patients, the kiosks ended up sitting idle and unused the majority of the day.

Kiosks were found to be utilized by less than 2% of patients[112] and the concept was eventually abandoned.

So, while not a panacea for all workflow or staffing problems, automation and new technology can help simplify and streamline work processes and reduce the "waste" of human talent when appropriately utilized.

4.5.2 STAFFING TO TAKT TIME

Optimum productivity depends on finding the right balance between staff and workload.

"Waste" of human talent in the form of *"muda"* or *"muri"* will occur when such a balance is not achieved or maintained; resulting in underutilized staff (or in the case of *"muri"* overworked staff), poor flow, and low employee morale.

Determining the appropriate number and type of staff needed is therefore critical to minimize the unnecessary "waste" of any human talent.

The number of staff needed can be balanced with workload by using TAKT time and cycle time.

TAKT time is the rate or speed at which work must be completed to service a patient or meet customer demand and is defined as:

112. Based upon an unpublished study of patient utilization of self checkin kiosk at several ambulatory clinics.

LEAN HEALTHCARE

$$\text{TAKT time} = \frac{\text{Available Work Time}}{\text{Customer Demand during available Work Time}}$$

where available time excludes lunch, breaks, meetings, and set up or change over time.

Cycle time, on the other hand, is the length of time required for a person or machine to actually complete a given job or task and can be calculated by observation, time study, estimation, or extrapolation (see appendix XI).

Once both of these numbers have been calculated, the resources needed to staff a department or activity can be determined.

The number of staff required equals cycle time divided by TAKT time as illustrated below:

$$\text{Staff needed} = \frac{\text{Cycle Time}}{\text{TAKT time}}$$

A typical after-hours walk-in clinic provides a good example of how TAKT time and cycle time can be used to determine the amount of staff required to run the clinic.

Assuming the after-hours clinic is staffed from 5 pm till 11 pm (a total of 6 hours), treats an average of 65 patients per night, and check-in at reception (cycle time) averages 5 minutes, nurse processing (cycle time) averages 10 minutes, and assessment and treatment (cycle time) by the physician takes 15 minutes; the TAKT time would be:

TAKT time = 320 minutes[113]/65 patients = 4.9 min/patient

113. Calculation of 320 minutes = 360 minutes – (10 minutes break)[114] – (30 minutes meal break)[114]

114. California Meal and Rest Break Law (2020), Gibbs Law Group
https://www.classlawgroup.com/employment/california-labor-law/meal-rest-break-laws/

Therefore, the staffing required in the after-hours clinic by position to meet a patient demand of 65 patients would be an average of 1 receptionist, 2 nurses, and 3 physicians (see table below):

Position	Patient Volume	Cycle Time (min)	TAKT Time (min)	Staff Needed
Clerk	65	5	4.9	1
Nurse	65	10	4.9	2
Physician	65	15	4.9	3

The number of staff required to run a department can be refined even further by looking at demand by hour, shift, or day of the week if there is significant variation from hour to hour, shift to shift, or day to day.

The Emergency Room provides a good example of how such variation in patient volume and TAKT time can be incorporated into the determination of the number of staff needed on a particular shift.

Assuming the Emergency Room treats an average of 150 patients on the day shift, 75 patients on the evening shift, and 50 patients on the night shift, and check-in at reception (cycle time) averages 6 minutes, nurse processing (cycle time) averages 18 minutes, and assessment and treatment (cycle time) by the physician takes 24 minutes; the TAKT time would be:

TAKT time =

Day	430 minutes[115]/150 patients =	3 min/patient
Eve	430 minutes[115]/75 patients =	6 min/patient
Night	430 minutes[115]/50 patients =	9 min/patient

115. 480 minutes – (10 minutes break x 2)[116] – (30 minutes meal break)[116] =430 minutes

116. California Meal and Rest Break Law (2020), Gibbs Law Group
https://www.classlawgroup.com/employment/california-labor-law/meal-rest-break-laws/

Therefore, the average staffing required in the Emergency Room to meet patient demand on the day shift would be 2 receptionists, 6 nurses, and 8 physicians; the evening shift 1 receptionist, 3 nurses, and 4 physicians; and the night shift 1 receptionist, 2 nurses, and 3 physicians (see table below).

TAKT time and cycle time can also be used to determine how work should be distributed between staff to reduce *"muri"* or overburdening and *"mura"* or unevenness in work.

Shift	Position	Patient Volume	Cycle Time (min)	TAKT Time (min)	Staff Needed
DAY	Clerk	150	6	3	2
	Nurse	150	18	3	6
	Physician	150	24	3	8
EVENING	Clerk	75	6	6	1
	Nurse	75	18	6	3
	Physician	75	24	6	4
NIGHT	Clerk	50	6	9	1
	Nurse	50	18	9	2
	Physician	50	24	9	3

Adequate staffing is frequently available in many departments and organizations; it's just not distributed appropriately to meet demand; resulting in bottlenecks, inefficiency, and delays.

A good example is an appointment center (see next page) that books patient appointments, maintains the physician master schedules, and processes physician schedule changes.

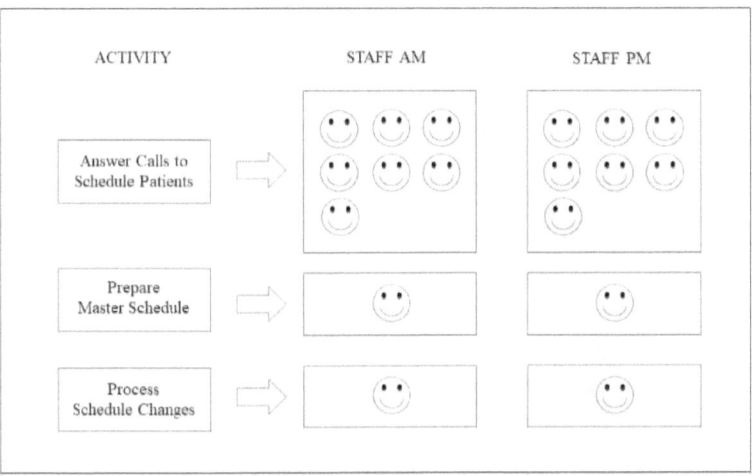

The call center depicted has a total of nine (9) staff with seven (7) dedicated to booking appointments, one (1) dedicated to processing schedule changes, and one (1) dedicated to master scheduling and receives an average of 630 calls per day (see distribution of calls below)

Hour	Call Volume
8 am – 9 am	110
9 am – 10 am	90
10 am – 11 am	80
11 am – noon	75
Noon – 1 pm	50
1 pm – 2pm	90
2 pm – 3 pm	50
3 pm – 4 pm	60
4 pm – 4:30 pm	25
Total	630

with each call averaging 4.5 minutes, receives an average of 70 schedule changes per day with each change averaging 3 minutes, and maintains the master schedule which requires an average of 7 hours per day.

The number of staff required to handle the volume of incoming phone calls per hour compared to the staff actually available is shown in the table below.

As seen in this table, the amount of staff available in the morning is insufficient to effectively handle the total number of calls received; while the amount of staff available in the afternoon exceeds the number of staff required to handle the afternoon volume of calls (a "waste" of human talent).

Hour	Call Volume	Cycle Time (min)	Available Minutes/Hr	TAKT Time (min)	Staff Needed	Variance to Actual
8 am – 9 am	110	4.5	60	0.54	8.3	(1.3)
9 am – 10 am	90	4.5	52.5	0.58	7.7	(0.7)
10 am – 11 am	80	4.5	52.5	0.65	6.9	0.1
11 am – noon	75	4.5	45	0.60	7.5	(0.5)
Noon – 1pm	50	4.5	45	0.90	5.0	2.0
1 pm – 2 pm	90	4.5	60	0.67	6.7	0.3
2 pm – 3 pm	50	4.5	52.5	1.05	4.3	2.7
3 pm – 4 pm	60	4.5	52.5	0.87	5.2	1.8
4 pm – 4:30 pm	25	4.5	30	1.2	3.7	3.3
Total	630					

Available minutes assume half the staff take their 15 minutes break between 9-10 and 10-11, half between 2-3, and 3-4 and half the staff take lunch between 11 – 12 and half between 12 -1.

Since the physician schedule changes can be handled anytime during the day, this disparity can be addressed by assigning the employee who processes the schedule changes in the morning to handling incoming calls.

This employee can then handle, along with one of the other employees who had been on the phones in the morning, all the schedule changes during the afternoon (see below).

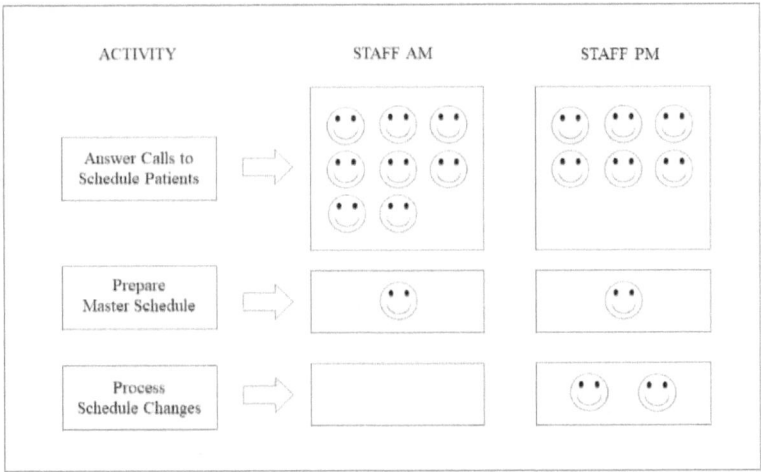

By shifting staff between these tasks, the gap between the number of staff needed to handle the incoming call volume during the morning is reduced or eliminated (see below).

Hour	Staff Needed	Original Gap	Gap After Adjustment
8 am – 9 am	8.3	(1.3)	(0.3)
9 am – 10 am	7.7	(0.7)	0.3
10 am – 11 am	6.9	0.1	1.1
11 am – noon	7.5	(0.5)	0.5

By redistributing staff in this way, the wait time for patients calling to book appointments can be reduced from an average wait of 13 minutes to an average wait of 2 minutes (see below); all without the need for

Staffing	Average Wait (min)	Max Wait (min)	% No Wait	% Wait < 5 min
Original	13.1	30.9	3%	26%
Redistributed	2.2	9.5	27%	83%

any increase in total staff.[117]

By comparing TAKT time to cycle time, appropriate staffing levels can be determined; better balancing staff with workload and helping to optimize productivity while minimizing the "waste" of human talent.

4.5.3   REDUCING DEFECTS

The defects or errors which occur in the delivery of healthcare are another cause of "wasted" human talent.

These defects or errors occur for a number of different reasons ranging from inadequate process design to poor communication and handoffs; resulting in rework or duplication of effort.

Examples of such rework or duplication of effort include:

- Repeat testing due to lost lab specimens

- Return of patients to the OR due to a retained foreign object

- Patient readmission to the hospital due to premature discharge

- Extended length of stay due to a medication error

The collection of specimens for the lab provides a good example of how defects or errors can result in the "waste" of human talent.

While most lab specimens that are collected are viable and can be used for testing and analysis, a certain percentage are not suitable or end up being unusable.

117. Analysis based on results of discrete event simulation using Extend simulation software.

Specimens may be unsuitable or unusable for a number of different reasons including insufficient volume, degradation of the specimen, and/or use of the wrong specimen collection tube.

Assuming a lab handles 700 specimens per day and has a reject/redo rate of 1%, then seven (7) specimens would need to be redrawn each day.

If these specimens came from different patients at different times throughout the day, then the phlebotomist would have to make multiple trips to the nursing floors to redraw the needed specimens.

Assuming it takes the phlebotomist six (6) minutes to walk to/from the floor each way/time a specimen needs to be redrawn and an average of seven (7) minutes to redraw each specimen, a total of 133 minutes or over 2 hours of phlebotomist time would be lost or "wasted" each day.

The impact of these errors, however, may extend beyond just the laboratory.

Delays in receiving critical test results may prevent timely diagnosis or treatment of patients' problems and extend patient stays by several hours or days; resulting in "wasted" bed and nursing hours.

Such defects and errors can be avoided by taking appropriate actions (see section 4.2); resulting in better utilization of available staff and helping to reduce the unnecessary "waste" of human talent.

4.5.4   IMPROVING FLOW AND LOAD LEVELING

Flow is the way work moves within and between departments.

When patients and work "flow", they move from one step in a process to the next without delay or interruption.

Delays and interruptions, however, are common throughout the entire healthcare delivery system because patients and work do not "flow" fluidly; resulting in the "waste" of human talent.

A good example of such waste is the preparation of patients for surgery.

Surgical site infections (SSI) represent one of the most common surgical complications reported in the U.S.; affecting an estimated 2% - 4% of all inpatient surgical patients.[118]

To reduce the risk of infection, the area around the surgical site must be properly prepped before the drapes are placed.

An antiseptic agent is typically applied to the surrounding tissue to kill potentially harmful microorganisms.

While Betadine has historically been used as an antiseptic agent because of its perceived efficacy, it requires a minimum of 10 minutes drying time before draping of the patient can begin.[119]

During the time the prep is drying, staff and surgeons must wait, often with few other tasks to do; wasting valuable staff, surgeon, and operating room time.

Different preps, such as Duraprep and Chloraprep, which are alcohol based have a much faster drying time than Betadine; requiring only 3 minutes to dry.[120]

118. Surgical Site Infections, Patient Safety Network, Agency for Healthcare Research and Quality, US Department of Health and Human Services, September 2019
https://psnet.ahrq.gov/primer/surgical-site-infections

119. Hemani, M. & Lepor, H. (2009). Skin Preparation for the Prevention of Surgical Site Infection: Which Agent is Best? *Rev Urol.* 2009 Fall; 11(4): 190–195.
https://www.ncbi.nlm.nih.gov/pmc/articles/PMC2809986/

120. 3M DuraPrep Surgical Solution, Commonly Asked Questions, Feb 2011
https://multimedia.3m.com/mws/media/820780/common-questions-duraprep-surgical-solution.pdf

By switching from Betadine to either Duraprep or Chloraprep, an operating room can save 7 minutes per case; without a significant increase in the risk of infection.[121, 122]

By taking actions such as this to eliminate delays and bottlenecks (see section 4.3) and improve "flow", productivity can be improved; helping eliminate or reduce the "waste" of human talent.

4.5.5 DEALING WITH POOR PERFORMERS

Hiring the best possible employees is a key responsibility of every manager.

However even the best managers can inadvertently hire the wrong candidate...one who turns out to be a poor performing employee.

Some of the attitudes and behaviors that typically lead to an employee being labelled as a poor or low performing employee include:

- Poor attendance

- Poor attitudes and/or work ethic

- Inadequate skills or competence

- Unacceptable work performance

- Low productivity

121. Pz et al. (2017).Prospective Randomized Trial Comparing the Efficacy of Surgical Preparation Solutions in Hand Surgery. *Hand* (N Y). 2017 May;12(3):258-264
https://www.ncbi.nlm.nih.gov/pubmed/28453340

122. Cozzoli et al. Chloraprep vs Povidone Iodine efficacy in the decrease of surgical site infection rate of post-operative patients. Penn State Hershey Nursing.
https://www.pennstatehershey.org/documents/1699942/10895543/GN2015July_Chloroprep/cf2665c8-0e87-438d-88ce-0c04644be299

Even though poor performing employees represent only about 3.7% of the workforce[123], their behaviors and attitudes can have a disproportionate impact on a department or organization.

Their poor attitudes and/or behaviors often lower the morale of other employees, waste management time and energy, generate extra work for other employees, and occupy a position that could be filled by a higher performing individual...all a "waste" of human talent (see appendix XII for more details on impact of poor performers).

While the best time to identify and address such performance issues is during the probationary period, performance issues often will not surface until after an employee has passed their probationary period.

> *Note: Almost a quarter of all employees put more effort into the job during the probation period than they do once they have secured the job.*[124]

This means that managers are often in the position of having to deal with employees' whose performance had previously been found to be "acceptable" and/or "competent".

Should this happen, their performance issue(s) must be dealt with immediately and without delay.

Actions which a manager may take to address an employee's performance issues include:

- Retraining

- Coaching

123. Performance Management Reference Materials, OPM.Gov, US Office of Personnel Management https://www.opm.gov/policy-data-oversight/performance-management/reference-materials/historical/dispelling-myths-about-poor-performers/

124. Lloyd, V. (2014). Twenty Percent Employees Fail to Pass Probation Period. *The HR Director*, May 14,2014 https://www.thehrdirector.com/business-news/employee-engagement/twenty-percent-employees-fail-to-pass-probation-period/

- Counseling

- Progressive discipline.

Such actions are effective in changing the behavior or performance of most, but not all, employees.

For those few employees that fail to show improvement or meet expectations (approximately 1.3% of all employees)[125], there are only two choices...tolerate their continued poor performance or terminate the employee.

Many managers, however, are reluctant to terminate an employee because of the effort, documentation, and stress involved; even though they know it is the right thing to do.

While the process for terminating an employee can be frustrating and time consuming, continuing to tolerate poor performance rather than terminating a poor performing employee is truly one of the greatest "wastes" of all.

4.6   "Treating" MOTION waste

The expenditure of effort is required to complete most tasks.

This expenditure of effort usually involves motion or movement...by either staff or machines.

If such motion or movement does not add value to a product, service, or

125. Meyer, A. (2016). Workers in Private Sector Are 3 Times More Likely to Get Fired Than Gov't Workers. *The Washington Free Beacon*. August 11, 2016
https://freebeacon.com/issues/workers-private-sector-3-times-likely-get-fired-govt-workers/

process (such as excessive or unnecessary walking); the energy and effort expended is essentially "wasted" and should be eliminated.

These "wasted" movements or motions can be reduced or eliminated by:

- Changing the physical layout or design of work areas to reduce distance traveled

- Using principles of 5S to organize work areas

- Simplifying or eliminating process steps

- Reducing or eliminating change over time

4.6.1   CHANGING WORK AREA LAYOUT

The physical layout of a work area should be configured to optimize "flow" and employee efficiency.

When work areas have not been properly laid out, employees end up walking further than necessary, reaching further than recommended, or bending or stooping more than is appropriate – all of which are forms of "wasted" motion.

The clinical laboratory provides a good example of how a poor physical layout of a work area can result in excessive walking and how reconfiguring the work area can help minimize unnecessary movement and motion.

The clinical laboratory uses a number of different instruments and equipment to perform analyses of blood and urine samples.

How and where these instruments or pieces of equipment are placed can affect how much wasted motion and walking is required.

LEAN HEALTHCARE

Traditionally laboratories have been laid out by department (i.e., hematology, chemistry, etc.) using long work benches to house the instruments and equipment (see example below).

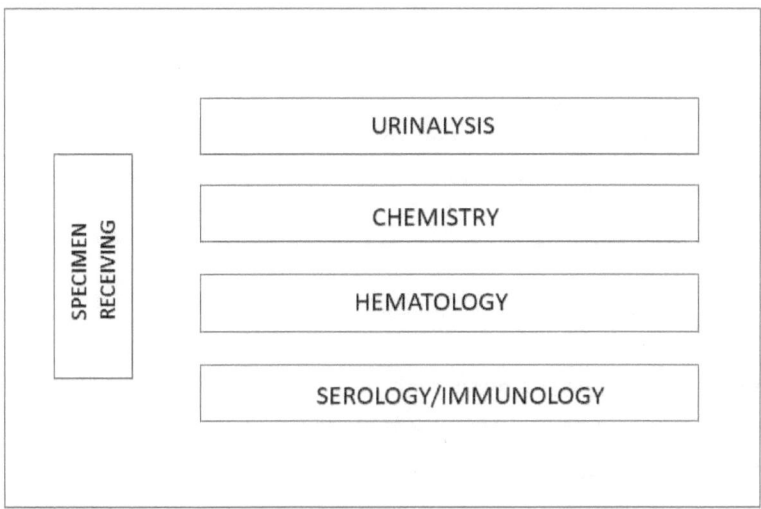

The linear configuration of these work stations often results in unnecessary motion and walking for the medical technologists when performing tests.

The hematology work station is where samples of blood are analyzed (see blowup of workstation in illustration on next page).

The most common tests performed in hematology are the coagulation and CBC tests.

To perform the coagulation test, the medical technologist must first centrifuge the sample to separate the plasma from its cellular components (i.e., RBC, WBC, platelets), then load the resulting sample into the analyzer, run the test, and print out and report the results.

To perform the CBC test, the medical technologist must load the CBC analyzer, run the test, then print out and review the results.

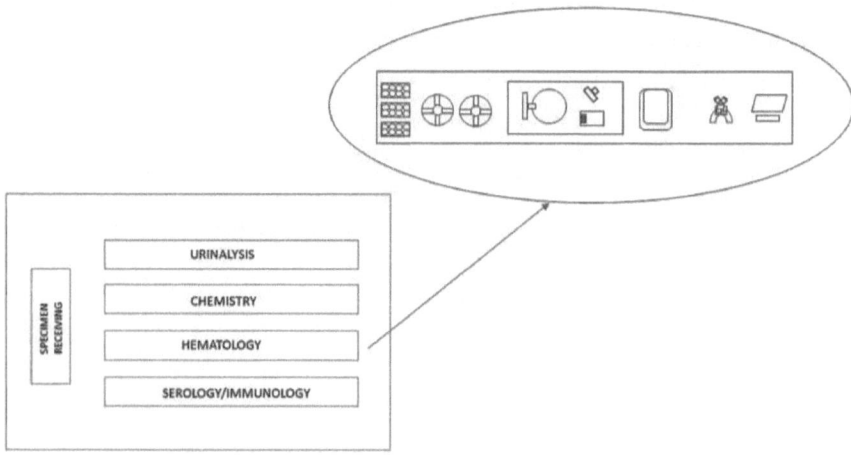

The medical technologist must then make a smear for any samples with positive results; which are then reviewed under the microscope and the results reported out.

A typical layout for a hematology work station is shown on the illustration below with instruments and equipment placed on the medical tech work bench in a linear configuration.

Assuming the medical technologist has to process 200 samples per day at this station (assuming an average batch size 5) they would travel back and forth 40 times; walking a total distance of approximately 800 feet.

10 feet

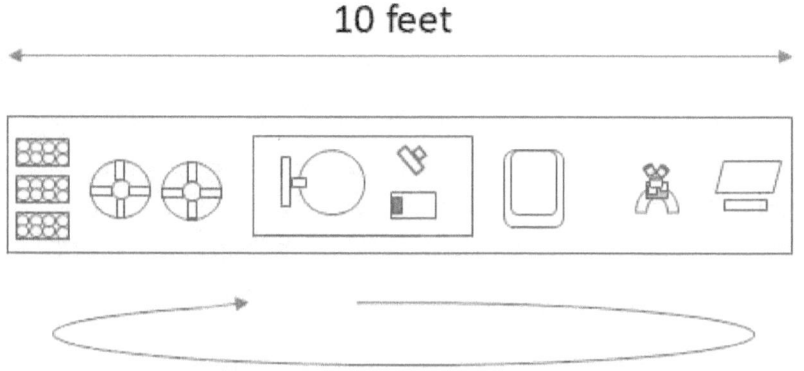

By changing the physical layout of the work station to a u-cell configuration (see below), the amount of distance the medical technologist would have to walk would be decreased approximately 500 feet; an almost 60% reduction.

5 feet

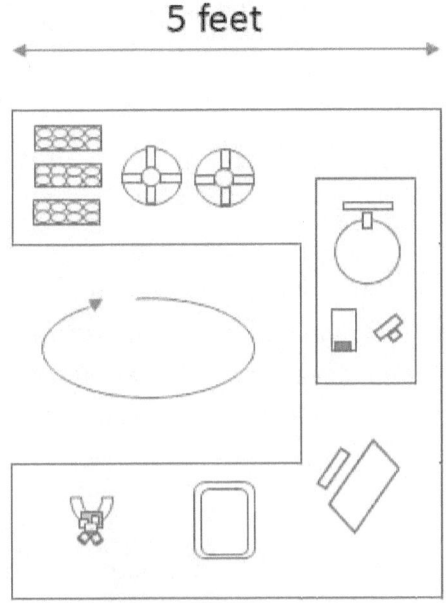

Making appropriate, and sometimes no more than minor, changes to department or workstation layout and design can help optimize workflow; reducing wasted motion and improving staff and clinician efficiency.

4.6.2   USE OF 5S TO ORGANIZE WORK AREAS

Besides being properly laid out, work areas also need to be properly organized to optimize employee efficiency and reduce or eliminate "wasted" motion.

Such "wasted" motion can be minimized by applying the principles of 5S.

5S is a mnemonic that stands for "sort", "set in order", "shine", "standardize", and "sustain", and represents a set of principles for organizing work areas to optimize staff and clinician efficiency and productivity.

These five (5) principles are defined as:

SORT

Sort through all items in a location and remove all unnecessary items from the location (i.e., outdated materials, broken equipment, redundant equipment, files on the computer, measurements which are no longer used).

SET IN ORDER

Determine, and then create, a specific location or spot for placement or storage of each item needed to perform the job (i.e., tools, equipment, supplies) which optimizes its retrieval and use for its function in the workplace.

SHINE

Clean, maintain, and keep the work area neat, orderly, and clear of clutter and potential safety hazards.

STANDARDIZE

Standardize the processes used to sort, order and clean the workplace.

SUSTAIN

Sustain the changes and improvements made to the organization of the work area.

The Central Distribution Department provides a good example of how poor organization of a work area can result in excessive "motion" (i.e., walking) and how 5S principles can help reduce such "waste".

Hundreds of supplies are typically stored in Central Distribution, ranging from housekeeping supplies to custom surgical packs, which are then distributed throughout the hospital as needed.

The demand for these items can vary significantly; with some items being pulled multiple times daily and some items being pulled only once every few months.

The placement of these items within Central Distribution relative to the distribution point can make a significant difference in the amount of walking needed to retrieve the items required.

The Central Distribution Department depicted on the next page is organized around an alphabetic placement of supplies; with items being stored in a location within the department based upon its name.

CENTRAL DISTRIBUTION LAYOUT

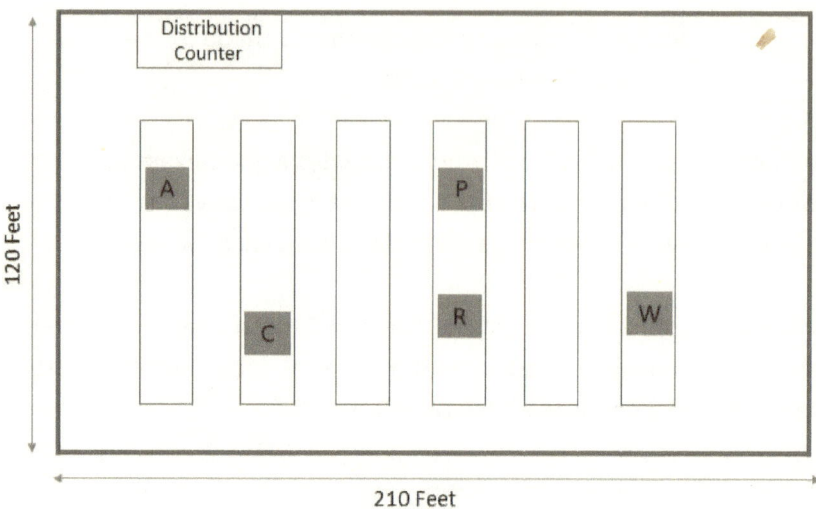

Assuming the weekly demand for each supply item shown below and the distance the storeroom worker must travel to retrieve the item each time it is requested, the storeroom worker(s) would have to travel approximately 125,400 feet per week to pull just these five (5) items.

Item	Distance Per Pull (ft)	Volume Pulled/Week	Total Distance (ft)
A	60	50	3,000
C	180	200	36,000
P	210	90	18,900
R	270	150	40,500
W	360	75	27,000
Total			125,400

The amount of distance that the storeroom worker(s) must walk can be reduced by applying the principles of 5S as follows:

SORT

Sort and rank supply items based on weekly usage into high demand and low demand items. Eliminate any supply items not requested in past year.

SET IN ORDER

Place highest demand supply items closest to distribution counter and low demand items furthest from distribution counter.

STANDARDIZE

Determine system for locating requested items in the storeroom and label shelves properly for easy identification and retrieval.

SHINE

Keep all items stored on shelves neat and orderly and clear of potential clutter or safety hazards.

SUSTAIN

Maintain improvements once implemented.

By reorganizing where items are placed in the storeroom (see illustration next page) and moving high volume items such as C, R, and W closer to the distribution counter, leaving item P where it is, and moving item A further from the distribution counter (see next page),

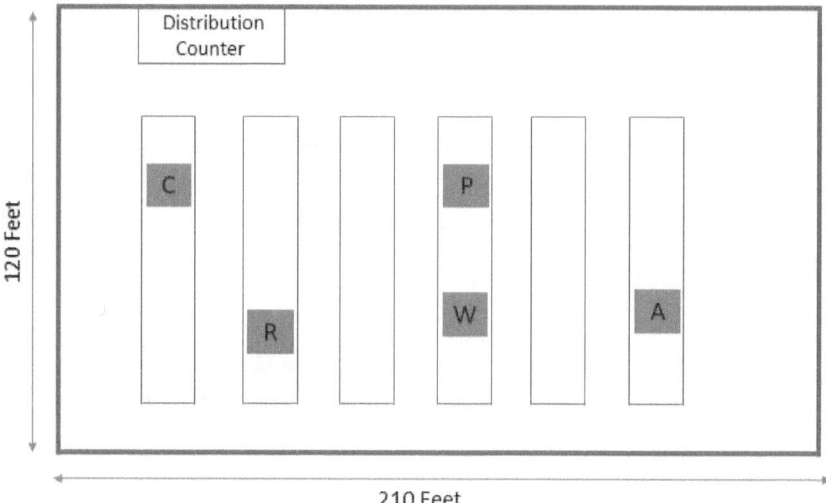

the distance walked by storeroom workers would be reduced from 125,400 feet to 96,150 feet; a reduction of unnecessary or "wasted" movement of 29,250 feet or 23% (see table below).

Item	Distance Per Pull (ft)	Volume Pulled/Week	Total Distance (ft)
C	60	200	12,000
R	180	150	27,000
P	210	90	18,900
W	270	75	20,250
A	360	50	18,000
Total			96,150

This would translate into a reduction of 1.5 hours of "wasted" movement per week (assuming the storeroom worker is walking at an average person's pace of 315 feet per minute).[126]

126. Based on Methods Time Measurement (MTM) standard of walking pace of 5.3 TMU per foot or 0.191 seconds per foot = 315 feet per minute.
Time saved = (125,400 ft – 96,150ft) / (315 ft/ min x 60 min)

By applying the principles of 5S to the organization of staff and clinician work areas, "wasted" motion can be reduced; resulting in improved staff and clinician efficiency and productivity.

4.6.3   SIMPLIFYING WORK PROCESSES

Work usually entails performance of a number of different tasks; each of which is comprised of a combination of basic motions (i.e., walking, reaching, etc.)

If the number of movements involved in a task (such as reaches, computer clicks, etc.) can be reduced, less energy, effort, and time is required to perform that task; eliminating "wasted" or unnecessary motion.

A good example of how the number of movements required to perform a task can be reduced is the physician order entry process.

Physician notes and orders are often manually typed or entered by the physician into an electronic medical record (EMR).

Some physician notes or orders (i.e., admission orders, discharge orders, etc.) can be lengthy; requiring extensive typing.

The number of characters (letters or number) that need to be typed by the physician can be reduced by simplifying the process and using a template or routine set of diagnosis specific notes, orders, or menus.

A template or order set can be pre-entered into an electronic health record and pulled up when needed by a physician; avoiding the need to type or enter the entire order into the EMR from scratch.

The orders can then be tailored to the individual patient by filling in the blank spaces on the template with patient specific dosages, frequency of treatment, etc., or by clicking the appropriate information or order to be included (see example below).

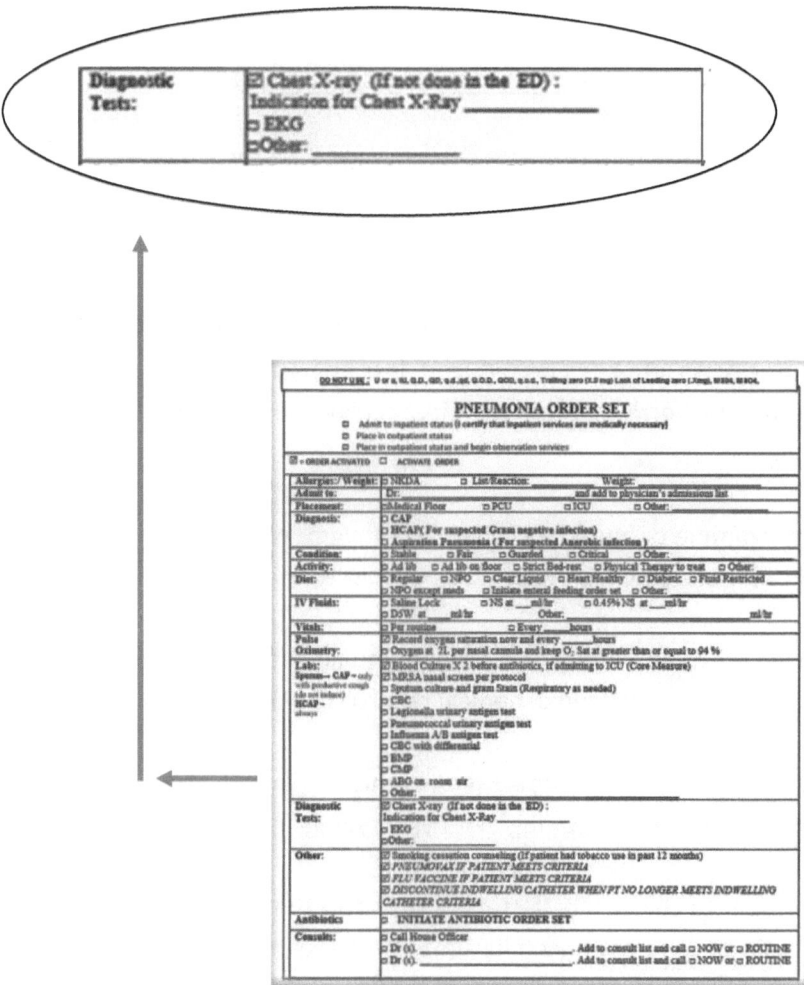

The use of order set menus at one hospital was found to reduce the time required to enter admission orders by 42%.[127]

127. Payne et al. (2003). Preparation and Use of Preconstructed Orders, Order Sets, and Order Menus in a Computerized Provider Order Entry System. *J Am Med Inform Assoc.* 2003 Jul-Aug; 10(4): 322–329. https://www.ncbi.nlm.nih.gov/pmc/articles/PMC181982/#bib17

At another hospital, the use of order sets increased the consistency in how patients were being treated and managed; reducing the pneumonia mortality rate by 56.5%.[128]

Simplifying work processes (such as with order sets and menus) can reduce "wasted" motion; leading to greater staff and clinician efficiency, productivity, and work quality/outcomes.

4.6.4   REDUCING SETUP OR CHANGEOVER TIME

A number of tasks that are performed in healthcare can-not be started until some setup or cleanup has been completed.

"Wasted" motion can be reduced if some or all of the steps required to cleanup or setup can be reduced.

A good example is the use of computers in healthcare organizations.

Employees and physicians in these organizations are dependent on computers to perform their jobs.

They are not, however, able to use the computer applications they need to access until they have logged in to the computer.

This login process which is designed to safeguard against unauthorized access to confidential patient, financial, or other organizational information often involves a two-step process.

The first step in this authentication process usually requires the entry of a physician or employee's user identification name or number followed by a second step typically requiring entry of a unique alpha numeric

128. Evidence-Based Care Standardization Reduces Pneumonia Mortality Rates and LOS, *Health Catalyst*. May 2018 https://www.healthcatalyst.com/success_stories/pneumonia-mortality-piedmont

user password.

The entry of a user ID and password is work that the employee or physician must perform as "setup" in order to access the screens or information they need to perform their "actual" work (i.e., entry of orders, filing of a work order repair request, etc.).

In most organizations the user IDs and passwords average about 8 – 10 characters [129] each in length; requiring 16 – 20 keystrokes each time a physician or employee has to login to their computer.

These keystrokes, which can be viewed as "wasted" motion, can be reduced by using other forms of authentication, such as smart card or biometric methodologies (i.e., fingerprint), which can be performed with the use of just one or two movements (i.e., swipe or touch).

By reducing the number of keystrokes or movements needed to log on, the setup time can be cut from an average of 8.4 seconds to just 1.1 to 2.6 seconds[130] each time authentication is required; resulting in greater efficiency, less user frustration, and less unnecessary or "wasted" motion.

4.7   "Treating" TRANSPORTATION Waste

Transportation of supplies, equipment, and patients within and between departments is often required in the delivery of healthcare.

This "movement" or transportation of people or things is often

129. Lampe, J. (2014). Beyond Password Length and Complexity. *General, Security, Management, Compliance, & Auditing*, January 6, 2014
https://resources.infosecinstitute.com/beyond-password-length-complexity/

130. Yakimov, V. (2011). Examining and comparing the authentication methods for users in computer networks and systems. Degree Project 10/27/11. Linnaeus University
http://www.diva-portal.se/smash/get/diva2:452090/FULLTEXT01.pdf

necessitated by poor workstation or department layout, isolated or siloed operations, or poor process design and controls.

Transporting or moving people or things, while needed to overcome such obstacles, does not add "value" to the services being provided; resulting in "wasted" energy, effort, and time.

This wasted movement or activity can be reduced or eliminated by:

- Integrating or centralizing services

- Decentralizing services

- Changing adjacencies or proximities of work areas

- Redesigning processes

- Using principles of 5S to organize work areas

- Handling items or patients as few times as possible

4.7.1   INTEGRATION OR CENTRALIZATION OF SERVICES

Transportation in most industries involves the movement of materials and supplies within or between work areas or facilities.

In healthcare, however, such transportation often involves more than just the movement of materials and supplies; it often involves the transportation of the facility's "customers" - the patient.

Transportation of patients is often required in healthcare as a result of many services being siloed due to organizational and bureaucratic impediments, incentives and politics, lack of physical proximities, or a physician-centric culture.

LEAN HEALTHCARE

Such transportation or movement of patients, which is considered "wasted" activity, can be reduced by integration of all or a portion of certain services.

A good example of how integration of all or a portion of certain services can reduce "wasted" patient movement is the preparation of patients for surgery.

Most hospitals require patients to be prepped several days prior to surgery.

This process usually requires patients to:

- See their surgeon for a preop physical

- Visit the lab to have their blood drawn

- See an anesthesiologist for a preop anesthesia assessment

- Go to Cardiology for an EKG (when indicated)

- Go to a preop education class (may be in person or virtual)

- Visit Admitting to be pre-admitted to verify payment sources and minimize registration time the day of surgery

Responsibility for these different functions frequently crosses organizational lines; creating bureaucratic, operational, and physical silos for performance of these activities.

Patients therefore often have to travel to different floors and areas of the hospital (see example on following page) to complete these pre-surgical tasks; "wasting" both their time and their energy.

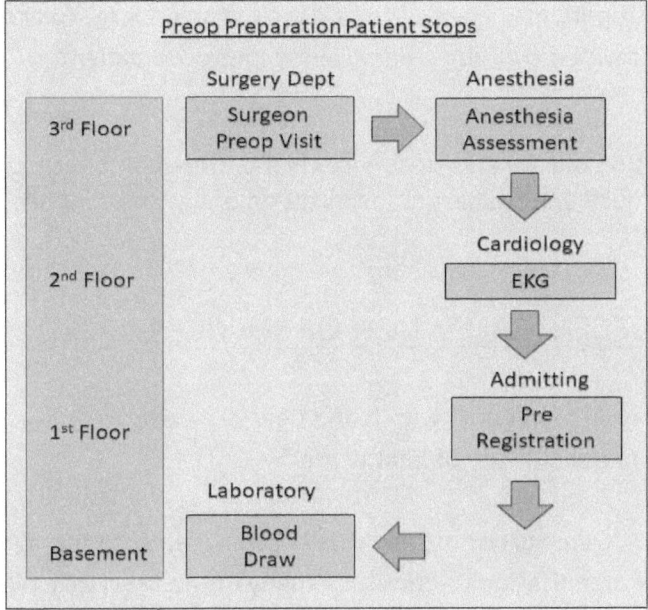

At many hospitals where such silos have been eliminated, most if not all, of these services have been incorporated into a centralized preop or patient assessment center (see illustration below).

Such centralization of services eliminates or reduces the need for patients to travel all around the medical facility in order to complete their surgical workup.

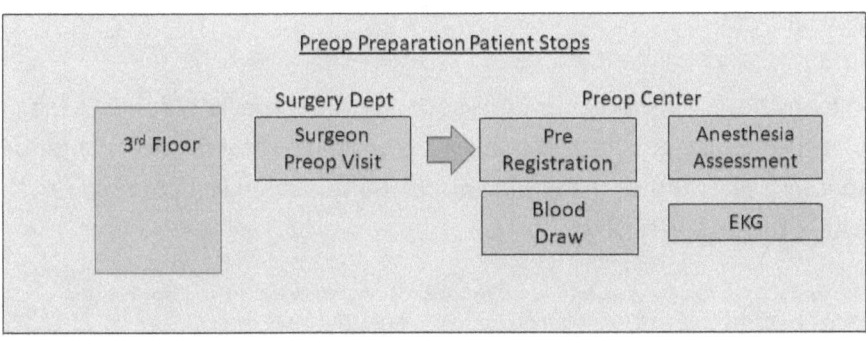

The result is patients have to spend less time and energy to access required services; creating a significantly improved patient care experience.[131, 132]

Centralization of care and/or services is therefore one alternative for helping reduce unnecessary transportation of patients, supplies, or equipment.

4.7.2   DECENTRALIZATION OF SERVICES

Transportation of patients within and between departments is often necessary in the delivery of healthcare.

The need to transport or move patients often stems from the practice of healthcare organizations centralizing many of their services in their quest to achieve economies of scale, to maintain manageable spans of control, and/or to optimize available facilities.

Such transportation or movement of patients is considered "wasted" activity and can be reduced by decentralization of all or a portion of certain services.

A good example of how decentralization can reduce unnecessary "wasted" patient movement or transportation is the delivery of specialty care.

In many healthcare organizations such as HMOs, specialty services (i.e., ophthalmology, podiatry, etc.) may be centralized at a medical center or specialty clinic rather than being dispersed to outlying clinics closer to where patients often live.

131. He et al. (2018). Improving patient flow and satisfaction: An evidence-based pre-admission clinic and transfer of care pathway for elective surgery patients. *Collegian* 25 (2018) 149 -156
https://www.collegianjournal.com/article/S1322-7696(17)30091-4/pdf

132. Pre-op testing center boosts efficiency, improves patient satisfaction, *Relias Media*, April, 1, 1997
https://www.reliasmedia.com/articles/56628-pre-op-testing-center-boosts-efficiency-patient-satisfaction

Patients are therefore forced to travel farther to access their specialty care when needed.

By decentralizing part or all of these services, care can be brought closer to the patient; reducing unnecessary or "wasted" motion or travel.

These specialty services may be decentralized by rotating specialty providers through outlying facilities or by using telemedicine technologies which enable specialty consultations at remote locations via video conferencing or other web-based applications.

Video consultations have been found in several studies to be an effective alternative to face to face consultations for diagnosis, treatment, and management of many medical issues.[133, 134]

Besides reducing the amount of travel required by patients, video consultation has also been found to improve overall patient satisfaction[133, 134], and reduce potential exposure to contagious illnesses from other patients seen in the physician's office.[135, 136]

By selectively decentralizing certain services, "wasted" or unnecessary transportation and travel can be reduced for patients...as well as in

133. Cheema, S. (2015). Video Visits: A closer look at patient satisfaction and quality of virtual medical care. *Applied Research Projects*. 30. University of Tennessee Health Science Center, Nov 2015 https://dc.uthsc.edu/cgi/viewcontent.cgi?article=1017&context=hiimappliedresearch

134. Buvik et al. (2018). Patient satisfaction with remote orthopaedic consultation by using telemedicine. A randomized controlled trial. *Journal of Telemedicine and Telecare*, July 24, 2018, https://journals.sagepub.com/doi/abs/10.1177/1357633X18783921?journalCode=jtta

135. Smith et al. (2020). Telehealth for global emergencies: Implications for Coronavirus disease (COVID-19). *J Telemed Telecare*. 2020 Mar 20 : 1357633X20916567 https://www.ncbi.nlm.nih.gov/pmc/articles/PMC7140977/

136. Kern, C. (2016). Virtual Care Helps Ease Bottlenecks and Spread of Disease During Flu Season. *Health IT Outcomes*, November 8, 2016 https://www.healthitoutcomes.com/doc/virtual-care-helps-ease-bottlenecks-spread-disease-during-flu-season-0001

many cases for physicians and other health care workers.

4.7.3   REDESIGNING PROCESSES

Patients are frequently transported to different areas of a medical center to undergo diagnostic or therapeutic procedures.

These procedures may include different imaging or surgical procedures.

Some of this transportation is unavoidable due to the size or availability of specialized equipment such as MRI machines or surgical robots.

Other types of tests or procedures, however, can be performed at the point of care; reducing the need to move and transport patients throughout the medical center.

A good example of how processes can be redesigned to reduce transportation "waste" is the performance of certain types of tests or procedures at the point of care.

Many surgical procedures are now performed in special procedure rooms rather than in hospital operating rooms.

The reason is that special procedure rooms are cheaper to run, often less regulated than operating rooms, and often provide greater flexibility in scheduling.

Special procedure rooms however are typically much smaller in size than an operating room (150 – 300 sq. ft. vs. 600 sq. ft.).

Podiatric and hand surgeries are often performed in special procedure rooms for these reasons.

Many of these procedures, however, involve the use of nails, plates, or screws; the placement and orientation of which often need to be verified during the procedure under fluoroscopy.

Most conventional c-arms, however, are too big to be used in a typical special procedure room, so patients in many facilities end up being transported to the Imaging Department to be x-rayed after the procedure to verify and document that the implanted nails, plates, or screws have been properly placed.

Some organizations have eliminated the need to transport these post-surgical patients to the Imaging Department by purchasing a Fluoroscan unit.

A Fluoroscan unit is a compact fluoroscopic imaging system that can fit in a special procedure room; allowing real-time imaging of the extremities (i.e., fingers, toes, hands).

By changing the process so that imaging can be performed in the special procedure room, the surgical process is streamlined; eliminating the need for "unnecessary" movement or transportation of the patient.

Transportation within healthcare, however, is not just limited to the movement of patients.

Large quantities of supplies must also be transported within and between areas or facilities primarily due to space limitations, bulk purchasing arrangements, and inventory management.

Since items are commonly received and stored at a location other than the point of use, transportation and multiple handling of these items is often required.

The amount of transportation required can sometimes be reduced by changing the process for how materials and supplies are received and distributed.

LEAN HEALTHCARE

A good example of how processes can be redesigned to reduce unnecessary transportation is the warehousing practices of some multi-hospital organizations.

One multi-hospital organization had all materials and supplies required for its hospitals delivered from each supplier weekly to a central warehouse in order to maximize price discounts.

The materials and supplies would then be unpacked and stocked on the shelves of the appropriate area in the warehouse.

When orders were received from each hospital, the appropriate items would be pulled from the warehouse stock and transported daily by truck to the hospital requesting the items.

After being unloaded from the truck, the items would be stocked in the hospital storeroom, and then distributed as needed to each administrative and/or clinical department in the hospital.

This process (see flowchart on next page) resulted in significant handling, transportation, and expense for each item needed.

Most suppliers offer drop shipping services where supplies can be delivered directly to an organization's individual hospitals or facilities; without loss of bulk purchasing discounts.

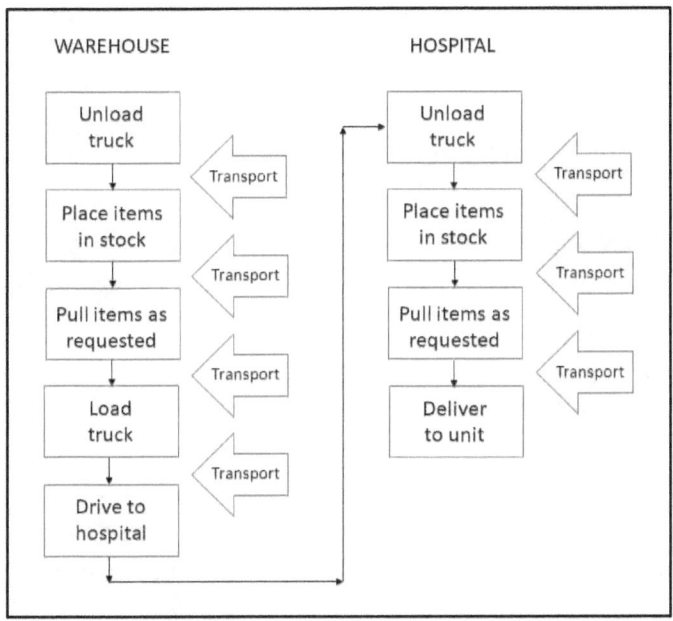

By changing the process (see below) to allow drop shipping of supplies

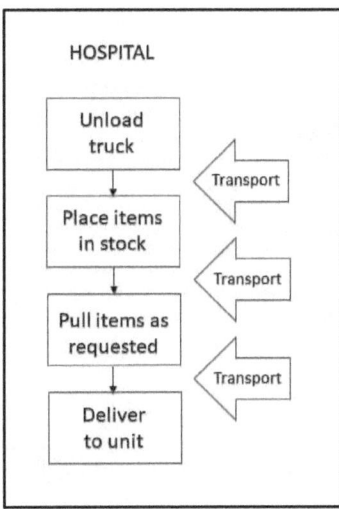

to individual hospitals and facilities within the organization, the amount of transportation and handling was significantly reduced; saving millions of dollars in warehousing, staffing, and trucking costs for the organization.[137]

4.7.5 USING PRINCIPLES OF 5S

One of the key principles of 5S (see section 4.6.2 for more details on principles) is that all the tools and materials that are required by an employee or physician are close at hand.

By placing such items close to where the work is being done allows unnecessary or "wasteful" transportation to be reduced or eliminated.

A good example of how the proximity of required tools can affect transportation waste is the printing at one lab of the labels used to identify the specimen containers for patients having their blood drawn.

At this lab, required labels were being printed on a shared printer located behind the phlebotomists' workstations (see below):

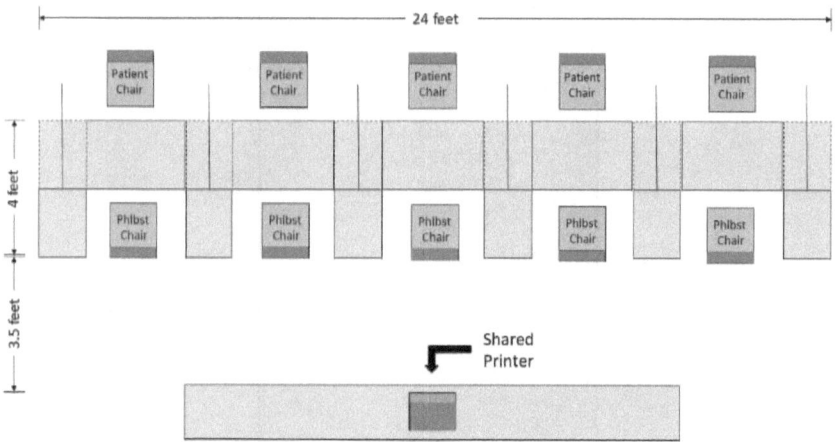

137. Results of unpublished analysis of one multi hospital purchasing, warehousing, and distribution practice.

Due to the placement of this printer, each phlebotomist was required to get up, leave their workstation, and retrieve the printed labels before they could begin drawing each patient's blood.

The need to repeatedly get up and leave their workstation to retrieve required labels was not only disruptive to workflow, but resulted in wasted time, energy, and motion.

Assuming a total of 600 patients per day, the five (5) phlebotomists would stand up/sit down a combined total of 600 times and average a collective 6,000 feet of travel/transportation.

By purchasing additional printers and placing them in closer proximity to each phlebotomist's workstation (see below), phlebotomists would no longer be required to get up and leave their workstations to retrieve patient labels; eliminating the need for transportation and saving a combined 1.2 hours per day.[138]

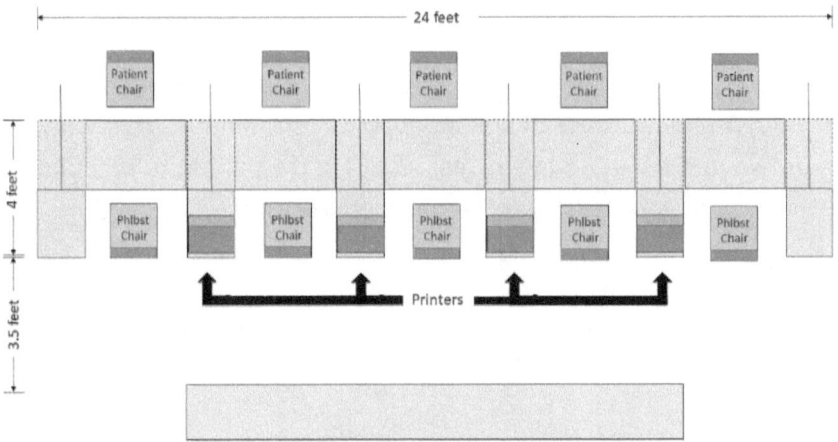

138. Assumes number of patients drawn per phlebotomist evenly split between the 5 phlebotomists, 2 phlebotomists walk 14 feet per round trip to retrieve printouts, 2 walk 8 feet, and 1 walks 6 feet using standard walking pace of 5.3 TMU per foot or 0.191 seconds per foot per Methods Time Measurement (MTM) and 5 seconds to standup, turn, and turn, sit down per trip per time study.

When appropriately applied, the principles of 5S can often reduce needless or "wasteful" transportation; saving time, energy, and unnecessary cost or delays.

4.7.6   HANDLE ONCE

Supplies and patients are often handled multiple times because of limited space, limited time, or poor processes.

Double or multiple handling can lead to "wasteful" and unnecessary transportation.

A good example of how "handling once" can reduce "wasteful" transportation is by looking at the way many patients' medical problems are handled by physicians.

When patients visit their physicians, especially their primary care doctor, they often present with numerous medical problems or complaints.

Many physicians, because of limited appointment time, address only one or two of the presenting issues; requiring the patient to schedule another visit to address their other problems or concerns.

This requires the patient to return to the physician office an additional time; resulting in unnecessary or "wasted" transportation or travel for the patient.

By taking a few extra minutes to address all of the patient's concerns at that one visit, the need for an additional patient visit would be avoided.

Not only does this eliminate an unnecessary trip for the patient (transportation), it also eliminates an unnecessary appointment in the physicians' schedule; helping improve both the physician's productivity and the availability of appointments for other patients wanting to see the provider.

The same concept applies to the handling of medical supplies.

A good example of how "handling once" can reduce transportation of supplies is the use of vaginal specula.

Vaginal specula are commonly used to perform pelvic exams.

Many clinics and hospitals purchase re-usable specula which must be sterilized prior to re-use.

Proper sterilization requires multiple handling, with specula often having to be transported to the Sterile Processing Department (SPD) for processing, sterilization, packaging, and then redistributed and transported back to the using practitioner.

By switching to disposable specula, many hospitals and clinics have been able to minimize the need for multiple handling and transportation of these specula.

Besides eliminating the need for multiple handling and transportation, the switch to disposables has been shown to reduce costs by up to 40% [139, 140] while helping to improve patient safety by reducing the risk of infection from improperly sterilized specula.

Unnecessary or wasted transportation and time can therefore be avoided by handling both patients or supplies just once (or if not possible as few times as absolutely necessary).

139. Phillips, P. (2000). Issues relating to disposable and reusable vaginal specula. MEDIDEX Nov 16, 2000
http://www.medidex.com/medical-devices/99-issues-relating-to-disposable-and-reusable-vaginal-specula.html

140. The Welch Allyn KleenSpec Advantage, Metal vs Disposable Vaginal Specula
https://www.welchallyn.com/content/dam/welchallyn/documents/sapdocuments/LIT/80018/80018670LITPDF.df

4.8   "Treating" OVERPRODUCTION Waste

A considerable amount of labor and supplies in healthcare are expended on admissions, appointments, and surgeries that are either inappropriate or unnecessary.

The expenditure of resources on such services or activities can be considered "overproduction" as they represent "wasted" time, effort, and energy.

Such overproduction in healthcare occurs as a result of misaligned incentives, variation in practice, pressure from patients and families, and/or breakdowns in the care delivery process.

Such overproduction or "wasted" activity can be reduced or eliminated by:

- Standardizing the criteria for surgery, admissions, and/or follow-up care using evidence-based criteria

- Aligning goals and incentives

- Implementing Just in Time

- Implementing production controls

4.8.1   STANDARDIZING CRITERIA

Variation in practice is commonly seen in the delivery of healthcare.

While some variation may be appropriate and reasonable based on a patient's age or medical condition; studies have found that as much as

80% of this variation is unwarranted[141] and can lead to overproduction and the provision of unnecessary treatment or care.

This unwarranted variation occurs as a result of differences in clinical training and knowledge, physician opinion or preference, and/or the availability of treatment options.

One way such unwarranted variation can be reduced or eliminated is by standardizing the criteria for providing high cost, high volume, or high-risk procedures, interventions, or care.

A good example of how standardization can reduce "overproduction" is the performance of screening mammograms for women.

There is significant variation among clinicians with respect to the ordering of screening mammograms for women; with many clinicians encouraging all women over 40 to have an annual screening mammogram.

Medical evidence, however, suggests that mammogram screening for most non high-risk women under 50, as well as for women over 74, is not effective in reducing the risk of breast cancer.[142]

In addition, this evidence suggests that the benefits of screening for women under 50 is outweighed by the potential risks associated with the incidence of high false positives and the performance of unnecessary biopsies, procedures, and treatment.[143]

141. Haughom, J. (2014). Clinical Variation in Your Medical Organization? *Health Catalyst*, June 16,2014 https://www.healthcatalyst.com/role-clinical-variation-medical-practice

142. Siu, AL (2016). U.S. Preventive Services Task Force. Screening for breast cancer: U.S. Preventive Services Task Force recommendation statement. *Annals of Internal Medicine* 2016;164(4):279–296.

143. Zinberg, J. (2015). Mammograms Are a Mixed Bag, Too much money is wasted on unnecessary breast cancer screenings, *US News and World Report*. July 23, 2015 https://www.usnews.com/opinion/economic-intelligence/2015/07/23/many-mammogram-breast-cancer-screenings-are-unnecessary

Evidence-based guidelines for mammogram screening were developed and distributed by the US Preventive Services Task Force. [144]

Within a year of their release, a 5% decline in the rate of "unwarranted" mammograms was seen nationally[145]; demonstrating the effectiveness of clinical guidelines in helping to minimize unwarranted variation along with the over production that accompanies it.

Similar findings were found at a number of healthcare organizations that developed standardized guidelines for diagnosis and treatment of various clinical problems.

At one organization, a set of clinical guidelines was developed and adopted called Choosing Wisely.

Patients being treated by physicians that followed all the guidelines had 14% fewer readmissions and 29% fewer complications than those patients whose physicians deviated from the guidelines; thereby avoiding needless care and lowering the cost of treatment, after adjustment for patient illness, severity, and complexity, by 7%.[146]

By simply standardizing clinical and administrative practices, "wasteful" variation can be reduced; improving quality while reducing over processing and the delivery of unnecessary care and services.

144. The United States Preventive Services Task Force (USPSTF) is an independent panel of experts in primary care and prevention appointed by the Department of Health and Human Services that systematically reviews the evidence of effectiveness and develops recommendations for clinical preventive services

145. Ruocco, M. (2016). Improving screening mammography: Perspective of a community radiologist. *Applied Radiology* Sep 2016
https://appliedradiology.com/articles/improving-screening-mammography-perspective-of-a-community-radiologist

146. Unnecessary medical tests, treatments cost $200 billion annually, cause harm. *Healthcare Finance* May 24, 2017, https://www.healthcarefinancenews.com/news/unnecessary-medical-tests-treatments-cost-200-billion-annually-cause-harm

4.8.2   ALIGNING GOALS AND INCENTIVES

The use of incentives has become increasingly popular as a way of focusing staff and physician efforts towards achievement of key quality, safety, and/or efficiency goals.

Such incentives are typically based on individual, team, or organizational performance and usually consist of some sort of financial reward or payout (i.e., bonus, profit sharing, etc.).

Such incentives, while intended to help achieve specific goals can sometimes have unintended consequences; resulting in overproduction and the delivery of unnecessary care.

A good example of how incentives can have unintended consequences, including overproduction, is pay for performance for cataract surgery.

An incentive program was implemented for the surgeons performing cataract surgery in a large capitated health care system to help improve patient access for surgery.

Each surgeon was expected to perform a minimum of 8 surgeries per assigned half day block (5 hours).

To help improve efficiency and access, each surgeon would receive a bonus for every surgery performed during the half day above that minimum threshold.

While the number of cataract surgeries performed per half day increased significantly following implementation of the incentive program, several unintended consequences resulted from implementation of the program.

Some of the surgeons had an insufficient volume of patients to consistently exceed the incentive threshold so they lowered the criteria for performing surgery to generate a sufficient volume of patients to receive incentive pay; resulting in overproduction and the premature performance of some surgeries.

Another unintended consequence was the impact on quality for one of the most "productive" surgeons, as evidenced by a jump in his rate of vitrectomies from less than 1% to 5%.[147]

These unintended consequences were addressed with some minor tweaking of the incentive program.

Similar findings were found in a study of surgical rates for Medicare cost patients where the surgeon got paid per surgery versus Medicare advantage patients where the surgeon got paid on a capitated basis.

The rate of cataract surgery for Medicare cost patients was found to be almost double that of the capitated Medicare advantage patients; reinforcing that incentive or compensation programs can lead to over production or the delivery of potentially unnecessary care or services.[148]

To avoid overproduction, it is therefore important that incentive or reimbursement programs be designed not only to be aligned with key goals, but also contain mechanisms for ensuring the program is not promoting unnecessary care nor compromising the quality of that care.

4.8.3   IMPLEMENTING JUST IN TIME

Supplies or services should be provided or delivered just in time to meet

147. Based on results of unpublished audit of vitrectomy rates from one hospital based ambulatory surgery center.

148. Study: Cataract surgery rate dropped under capitation, *Healio Ocular Surgery News*, January 4, 2006, https://www.healio.com/ophthalmology/cataract-surgery/news/online/%7Be58d6727-64be-42df-941a-0cda237de0fc%7D/study-cataract-surgery-rate-dropped-under-capitation

the patient's or client's need.

Delivering or providing a supply or service before it is requested or needed by a patient can result in overproduction and the delivery of unnecessary services or care.

A good example of how providing care and services "just in time" can reduce overproduction is the filling of outpatient prescriptions.

Following implementation of a new electronic medical record (EMR) order entry system in one integrated healthcare system, the clinic physicians automatically sent all prescriptions down to the facility's pharmacy to be filled.

The intent was that by the time the patient arrived in the pharmacy, their prescription would be ready to be picked up; saving the patient time and providing the patient with an exceptional service experience.

While there was a reduction in wait time for patients to pick up their prescriptions; the benefits were offset by a large number of prescriptions never being picked up and having to be restocked; resulting in a waste of limited manpower.

Such waste can be minimized by waiting to provide any supplies or services until actually requested or needed by patients, staff, or physicians and then providing them "just in time".

4.8.4   IMPLEMENTING PRODUCTION CONTROLS

Overproduction is a common problem for Dietary Departments in hospitals.

Meals are often prepared for patients that are either unneeded or go uneaten.

Hospitals have been found to have a rate of wasted meals 2 to 3 times higher than that found in other food service sectors.[149]

Reasons for such overproduction include changes in patient condition, changes in patient dietary requirements, and changes in patient status (i.e., patient discharged from the hospital).

The number of meals that are "wasted" can be reduced by implementing appropriate management and production controls.

A good example of how such controls can help reduce "wasted" meals is provided by the actions taken by one hospital which had a rate of "wasted" meals 23% below that of similar hospitals.[150]

One of the most important production controls implemented by this hospital to help reduce the volume of "wasted" meals was to routinely forecast and monitor meal demand so as not to "overproduce" the number of meals needed.

Such forecasting was done using historical data and making adjustments based on current census.

Another important production control was improving communication between the nursing units and the dietary department.

Timely communication from the nursing units to the kitchen about changes in patient status, dietary requirements, or availability helped prevent overproduction and avoided the preparation and delivery of incorrect, unwanted, or unneeded patient meals.

149. Gunders, D. (2019). Hospital Wastes A Third Less Food After This One Change. *Forbes* Feb 18,2019
https://www.forbes.com/sites/danagunders/2019/02/18/hospital-wastes-a-third-less-food-after-this-one-change/#469996bd18c4

150. Reducing Food Waste in Irish Healthcare Facilities, Green Healthcare
https://www.epa.ie/pubs/advice/green%20business/Reducing-food-waste-in-Irish-healthcare-Facilities-foodwaste-guidance-booklet-reduced-size.pdf

Over-control of the production process can also lead to overproduction.

Hospitals historically produce food in bulk and serve it to patients at predetermined times; even though the patient may not be available or hungry...resulting in many meals going uneaten or "wasted".

The restrictions on when meals could be prepared were loosened at one hospital with implementation of an "on demand" or "room service" system.

This "production" change allowed patients the flexibility of having their meals ordered, prepared, and delivered at a time of their choosing; resulting in a 30% reduction in the number of meals per day that ended up being "wasted".[151]

By implementing appropriate management and production controls, the potential for overproduction can be reduced or eliminated; helping to avoid "wasting" costly labor and supplies.

4.9 "Treating" OVERPROCESSING Waste

Patients may receive care or services that are unnecessary, duplicative, or of limited value.

The expenditure of resources on care or services of limited value may be considered "overprocessing" and seen as "wasteful".

Such "overprocessing" in healthcare may occur as a result of malpractice concerns, workload, or provider practice.

Some of the actions that can be taken to minimize overprocessing include:

151. Three Tips to Reduce Hospital Food Waste, Head Green Guru, Green Impact
https://www.greenimpact.com/best-practices-and-tools/three-tips-to-reduce-hospital-food-waste/

- Reassessing the value of each step in the process

- Standardizing or using clinical guidelines

- Starting with a conservative approach

- Hardwiring changes

4.9.1   REASSESS THE VALUE OF EACH PROCESS STEP

Processes consist of a number of different steps.

Each step in a process should exist to add "value" to the customer or patient experience.

Many processes in healthcare, however, have been designed for the added convenience of the provider, rather than the added value for the patient...resulting in overprocessing and "waste".

The preop anesthesia process for cataract surgery at one hospital provides a good example of how process design can lead to overprocessing.

According to various regulatory agencies, a preop anesthesia evaluation must be performed immediately prior to surgery for each patient who receives general, regional or monitored anesthesia care (MAC).

This assessment typically involves an assessment of patient vitals, airway, anesthesia risk (ASA), and medical history, along with documentation of the anesthesia provider's plan of care.

At one hospital this preop anesthesia assessment was performed the week prior to surgery in order to "streamline" the anesthesiologists' workload the day of surgery.

The anesthesia provider would then perform a "quick" reassessment of each patient the day of surgery as prescribed by regulatory requirements.

Approximately 12% of the surgical patients seen in the preop anesthesia clinic at this medical center (1,500 of 12,000 per year) were cataract patients.

Cataract surgery is considered a low risk procedure involving use of topical anesthetics (and possibly sedation) and typically does not require a lengthy anesthesia workup.

The need for all cataract patients to be seen prior to the day of surgery was evaluated and the practice discontinued after determining that performing two anesthesia assessments on these patients was actually of limited value and constituted "overprocessing" of the patient.

By eliminating the preop anesthesia visit for all cataract patients the hospital was able to reduce an unnecessary visit for the patient and reduce the workload in the anesthesia clinic; without affecting the quality of care or surgical outcomes.

Validating the value of each step in a process and eliminating those that do not provide "added" value can reduce or prevent overprocessing and all its associated "waste".

4.9.2   STANDARDIZE

Referrals from primary care physicians to specialists happen routinely in healthcare.

In many instances, such referrals are made even when the primary care physician can successfully manage the patient's problem.

Such "overprocessing" can be minimized by developing clinical guidelines and standardizing the workup and treatment required before a referral can be made.

A good example is the management of plantar fasciitis.

Plantar fasciitis is an inflammation of a thick band of tissue that connects the heel bone to the toes.

Referral of a patient diagnosed with plantar fasciitis to a podiatrist is common, even though initial treatment (i.e., nonsteroidal anti-inflammatory drugs, orthotics, etc.) can be provided by the primary care provider and is effective for 90 percent of patients.[152]

Many organizations have addressed this practice by establishing referral guidelines (see example on next page) which require workup and specific treatment before authorizing referral of a patient to podiatry.

If the patient is found to be unresponsive to the recommended treatment, the primary care provider is then encouraged to refer the patient to Podiatry for further evaluation and treatment.

Such guidelines were developed for plantar fasciitis by the podiatry department in one multi-specialty medical group.

Following development and distribution of these guidelines, the total number of plantar fasciitis referrals dropped by over 70%.[153]

By developing clinical guidelines which standardize the workup and treatment required before a referral can be made; overprocessing and

152. Fullem, B. (2016). A Guide to Conservative Care for Plantar Fasciitis. *Podiatry Today* October 21, 2016 https://www.podiatrytoday.com/guide-conservative-care-plantar-fasciitis

153. Based on results from unpublished study of referral rates in one multi-specialty medical group.

PLANTAR FASCIITIS
Referral Guidelines

Eligibility
- Pain on the plantar aspect of the heel
- Unilateral
- Pain is most severe in the am or after prolonged sitting
- Becomes worse if barefoot

Differential Diagnosis
- Stress fx of the calcaneum
- Inflammatory arthropathy
- Retrocalcaneal bursitis or insertional achilles tendinitis
- Tarsal tunnel syndrome

Information Required for Referral
- Detailed history of the pain
- Occupational history
- Associated back or joint pain
- Any history of trauma to the heel
- Any treatment used (i.e. orthotics, steroids, etc.)
- Examination : exact location of the pain
- Rule out retro calcaneal bursitis, tarsal tunnel syndrome by localization of the pain

Actions Required Prior to Referral
- Weight bearing foot x-rays
- Optional : ultrasound to identify thickening in plantar fasciitis

Suggested Primary Care Management
- Consider orthotics
- Consider physiotherapy
- Analgesics and anti-inflammatory medications
- Ultrasound guided steroid injections
- This is often a self-limiting condition and will improve in 6 to 24 months from onset without specific treatment

Referral Indicated
Continuous pain despite non-operative management

the unnecessary "waste" of specialist time, knowledge, and skills can be reduced while ensuring the patient receives the appropriate treatment needed.

4.9.3   START WITH A CONSERVATIVE APPROACH

There are often a number of different options that are available for treatment of a given medical problem.

These treatment options may range from conservative approaches such as changes in diet, use of medicines or injections to aggressive approaches such as surgery.

One way to avoid overprocessing is by starting treatment with one or more of the conservative or non-invasive approaches before starting any of the more aggressive or invasive approaches.

A good example is the treatment of carpal tunnel syndrome.

Carpal tunnel syndrome is a very common problem that affects approximately four (4) percent of the general population in the United States.[154]

Carpal tunnel syndrome is a condition characterized by numbness, tingling and other symptoms in the hand and arm and is often associated with repetitive hand motions and the compression of the nerve in the carpal tunnel.

There are a number of different approaches for treating carpal tunnel ranging from wrist splinting, nonsteroidal anti-inflammatory drugs, corticosteroid injections to physical therapy and/or surgery.

The effectiveness of these treatments varies considerably.

154. Carlson et al. (2010). Current options for nonsurgical management of carpal tunnel syndrome. *Int J Clin Rheumtol* 2010 Feb; 5(1): 129–142.
https://www.ncbi.nlm.nih.gov/pmc/articles/PMC2871765/

The more conservative approaches such as wrist splinting and nonsteroidal anti-inflammatory drugs show improvement for about 40 percent of patients treated.[155]

The more intensive and invasive (and more costly) approaches such as physical therapy and surgery show improvement for about 90 percent of those treated.[156, 157]

Given the success rate of these more conservative treatments, a phased approach that starts with conservative treatments and progresses to the more intensive/invasive treatments (in the absence of improvement) can ensure patients receive the most appropriate treatment for their problem; thereby avoiding overprocessing and its associated "wastes".

4.9.4   HARDWIRING CHANGES

Change has been occurring in many areas of healthcare.

These changes have ranged from the availability of new medicines and treatment options to the availability of new equipment and technologies.

Historical practices and procedures however can sometimes persist even after these changes have been adopted or implemented; resulting in overprocessing and "waste".

155. Rozmaryn, L. (1997). Carpal tunnel syndrome: A comprehensive review. *Current Opinion in Orthopedics*, 1997, 8:IV 33-43
https://www.leohanddoc.com/pdf/carpal-tunnel-syndrome-a-comprehensive-review.pdf

156. Carpal Tunnel Syndrome: Outlook/Prognosis, Cleveland Clinic
https://my.clevelandclinic.org/health/diseases/4005-carpal-tunnel-syndrome/outlook--prognosis

157. Fernandez-de-las-Penas et al. (2015). Manual Physical Therapy Versus Surgery for Carpal Tunnel Syndrome: A Randomized Parallel-Group Trial. *The Journal of Pain*, Vol16 No 11, 2015, pp 1087-1094
http://atmis.pl/wp-content/uploads/2017/12/J-Pain-2015-16-11-1087-1094.-Manual-therapy-vs.-surgery-for-CTS.pdf

A good example is the process used in many large medical offices for notifying the module nurse that a patient has checked in and is ready to be processed.

The patient registration area for many large medical offices is often centralized and physically separated from module waiting rooms and patient intake areas.

A piece of paper, which would be dropped in a slot in the wall of the waiting room, would often be used to communicate to module nurses that the patient had checked in and was ready to be processed.

The use of this form of notification would often be so integrated into module workflow, that staff would continue to rely on paper communication even after electronic alternatives have been "implemented"; resulting in overprocessing and unnecessary "waste".

Habits, which make up over 40% of most people's daily activities,[158] help routinize employee behaviors and form the foundation of many organizational work processes.[159]

The habits associated with any old routines must be "broken" before they can be replaced by the new work processes or routines.

Breaking these old habits can be difficult and requires:

- A clear understanding by staff and clinicians of what behaviors are to change, what behaviors are to continue, and why

158. Sherman, R. (2013). Hardwiring Nurse Practice Changes. *Emerging RN Leader* August 1, 2013
https://www.emergingrnleader.com/nursing-practice-changes/

159. Duhigg, C. (2012). The Power of Habit, Why We Do What We Do in Life and Business. Random House, 2012
http://fop86.com/The%20Power%20of%20Habit/The%20Power%20of%20Habit.pdf

- Simulation and testing of new processes and associated behaviors before actual transition

The new habits can then be "hardwired" to replace the old habits through repetition, observation, and reward and reinforcement; helping to avoid overprocessing and its associated "waste".

4.10 "Treating" waste CHECKLIST

Waste is commonly found in the delivery of healthcare.

A number of "treatments" or mitigation strategies were discussed to reduce or eliminate such waste (see matrix on next page).

Successful "treatment" is important for improving the quality, efficiency, affordability, and safety of healthcare.

In medicine, it is far better to prevent the occurrence of illness than to treat it.

The same is true for organizational "waste".

It is far better to "prevent" the occurrence of organizational "waste" than to have to "treat" it after the fact.

A number of strategies and tactics are available for "preventing" such waste.

Having examined the most common strategies and tactics that can be taken to *treat* "waste", the next step is to look at what actions or steps can be taken to *prevent* "waste" from even occurring in the first place.

STRATEGIES AND TACTICS

Strategies and Tactics	Defects	Waiting	Over production	Overprocessing	Motion	Transportation	Inventory	Human Talent
Poka-Yoke/error proofing	■	■			■			■
Jidoka/andons	■	■			■			■
Reduce/improve handoffs	■	■		■	■			■
Standardized work/protocols	■	■		■	■			■
5S	■	■			■			■
Checklists	■	■		■	■			■
Reduce variation	■	■	■	■	■			■
Automation/new technology	■	■		■	■			■
Inservicing	■	■		■				■
Channelling	■				■	■	■	■
Shaping demand		■					■	■
Load leveling		■						■
Shifting demand		■						■
Reducing demand		■						■
Process redesign	■	■		■	■			■
Eliminate process steps	■	■		■	■			■
Combine rearrange steps	■	■		■	■			■
Perform steps in parallel		■						■
Reduce turnover/SMED		■			■			■
Increase capacity		■						■
Redistribute staff/machines		■						■
Cross train staff/machines		■						■
Add additional staff/machines		■						■
Implement one piece flow	■	■				■	■	■
Utilize small piece processing	■	■				■	■	■
Pool resources		■				■	■	■
Just in Time		■	■			■	■	■
Kanban			■			■	■	■
Staff to tak time		■						■
Centralization		■			■	■	■	■
Decentralization		■			■	■		■
Address poor performers	■							■
Goal/incentive alignment			■	■				■
Conservative approach					■			■
Change physical layout		■			■		■	■
Production controls/Forecasting			■			■	■	

■ Represents potential "treatment" options

PREVENT

Preventing Waste

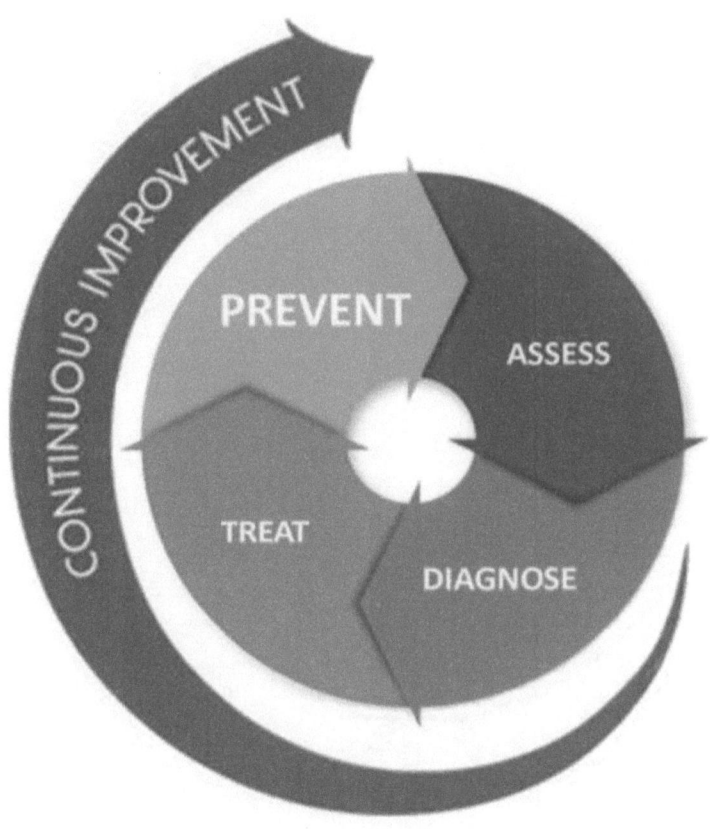

CHAPTER 5
How to Prevent Waste

5.1   An Ounce of PREVENTION...

Preventive care has become a critical part of the plan for management of the health and wellness of many patients.

The increased emphasis placed on prevention has stemmed from studies which show that preventive care can help patients avoid development of much more serious medical conditions or illnesses.[160, 161]

The same applies to business processes, procedures, and systems.

The "health" of a department or organization can be enhanced or maintained by taking certain preventive steps to reduce the risk of "waste".

There are a number of tools available to help prevent waste from infecting or impairing business processes before they happen.

Some of the prophylactic approaches available for preventing "waste" include:

- Conducting a Failure Modes and Effects Analysis (FMEA)

160. Preventive Care, Wikipedia
https://en.wikipedia.org/wiki/Preventive_healthcare

161. Guide to Evidence Based Prevention, Health Policy Institute of Ohio, December 2013
https://nnphi.org/wp-content/uploads/2015/08/GuideToEvidence-BasedPrevention.pdf

- Error proofing processes (*Poka-yoke*)

- Performing timely and appropriate preventive maintenance

- Conducting simulations or drills

5.2   Failure Modes and Effects Analysis

Processes often evolve and change over time.

As they evolve and change, weaknesses can develop which can cause potential problems or "failures".

Identifying and mitigating these potential weaknesses or "failures" can help prevent "waste" from occurring in the process.

Failure Modes and Effects Analysis (FMEA) is one approach that can be used to help identify such weaknesses or "failure modes".

Using a team of staff and/or clinicians familiar with the process being evaluated, the team conducts a systematic review of each step of the process asking:

- What could go wrong?
  (in order to identify failure modes)

- Why would the failure happen?
  (in order to identify the causes of a failure)

- What would be the consequences of each failure?
  (in order to identify the effects of such a failure)

- What can be done to prevent such failures from happening?
  (to identify actions which could be proactively taken)

LEAN HEALTHCARE

A good example of how Failure Modes and Effects Analysis can be used to reduce the risk of error is with cataract surgery.

At one hospital, even though it had never experienced a cataract related "never event", a team of staff and physicians was chartered to perform an FMEA with the mission of identifying any potential risks or failures related to patient safety.

The team reviewed the entire process for cataract surgery as part of the FMEA asking:

- What could go wrong?

- Why would the failure happen?

- What would be the consequences of each failure?

- What can be done to prevent such a failure from happening?

One of the team's findings was that over time, as the number of cases per half day increased, their practice for handling interocular lens (IOL) had changed; with the lens for more than one patient being kept in the operating room during surgery.

While more efficient, this practice was felt to provide the opportunity for the interocular lens (IOL) for the wrong patient to be accidentally pulled and implanted in a patient during the surgery.

To reduce the risk of the wrong IOL being implanted, the team recommended that they return to the practice of having only one patient's IOL in the OR at a time.

As a result, the surgical process was changed to reflect the recommendation of the team; helping to "prevent" potential insertion of the wrong lens during surgery and the occurrence of a *never event*.

By trying to identify potential "failure points" before a problem has even occurred, FMEA can help "prevent" or avoid problems from actually occurring that affect the quality, safety, or cost of patient care.

5.3   Error Proofing Processes

Error proofing or *poka-yoke* is another common approach used to help "prevent" unnecessary waste.

Error or *mistake* proofing involves designing a product or process to "prevent" a mistake from inadvertently happening by use of physical, mechanical, and/or design controls (also see section 4.2.1).

Such controls are commonly found in healthcare settings; especially as a mechanism for helping to ensure patient safety.

Some examples of the physical, mechanical, and design controls used to protect patient safety include different shaped connectors for hooking up medical devices to medical gases, devices that turn X-ray machines off whenever roentgen levels exceed acceptable levels, and child proof bottles with twist caps that need to be depressed and twisted before they can be removed.

While use of mechanical, physical, or design controls are the most effective approach for preventing errors, use of such controls may not always be feasible.

In those cases, procedural controls may need to be utilized to minimize the risk of error.

A good example of procedural controls is the universal protocol; a procedure that has been implemented in many operating rooms to prevent the occurrence of a "never event", such as wrong side, wrong site, or wrong patient surgery.

The universal protocol consists of three key elements:

- **Pre-procedure verification** process to address missing information or discrepancies before the start of the procedure

- **Pre-surgical site verification and marking** to ensure the correct side and site are clearly marked

- **Timeout** or **pause** immediately prior to incision to explicitly confirm **1)** the identity of the patient, **2)** what procedure is planned, and **3)** the correct site of surgery.

A checklist such as that shown on the next page can be used to aid surgeons and staff in completing each step of this procedural control process.

At one hospital, the rate of wrong side, wrong site surgeries were reduced by almost 75 percent following implementation of the universal protocol;[162] demonstrating that while not fool proof, procedural controls can help "prevent" errors.

Many problems or errors can therefore be "prevented" or avoided by error proofing processes with the appropriate mechanical, physical, design, or procedural controls.

162. Based on results from unpublished study of never events in one mid-sized community hospital reporting reduction in never events from 1 in 10,000 cases to 1 in over 36,000 cases.

UNIVERSAL PROTOCOL CHECKLIST

Pre Procedure Verification

Patient Identification (need 2):
- ❏ Name/DOB
- ❏ Verbal with patient/family
- ❏ Other (i.e. Medical record number

Procedure Verification:
- ❏ Procedure confirmed with patient or designee
- ❏ Consent for procedure signed
- ❏ Relevant documentation completed, reviewed, signed
- ❏ Clinical indications for procedure

Marking

Operative Site Marked:
- ❏ Yes
- ❏ No

Time Out

Prior to procedure:
- ❏ All team members present
- ❏ Correct patient identified
- ❏ Agreement on procedure
- ❏ Correct side and site   N/A
- ❏ Correct patient position
- ❏ Availability of correct implant   N/A
- ❏ Availability of correct equipment   N/A

5.4 Preventive Maintenance

A considerable amount of equipment, medical devices, and machines are used in the delivery of healthcare.

Unplanned breakdown of these items can disrupt workflow and cause problems, delays, and frustration for patients, staff, and physicians.

Breakdown of these items can often be avoided if "preventive" maintenance is performed on them at appropriate intervals.

Four methods are commonly used to determine when preventive maintenance is required.

These methods are:

- **A calendar-based schedule**

  which uses the time elapsed since the last date the unit was serviced to determine when the next preventive maintenance service should be performed

- **A usage-based schedule**

  which uses volume or usage information to determine when the next preventive maintenance service should be scheduled

- **A predictive-based schedule**

  which uses historical information and events to identify when preventive maintenance services should be scheduled

- **A prescriptive maintenance-based schedule**

  which uses historical information and events along with machine learning software to identify when preventive maintenance services should be scheduled

A good example of how preventive maintenance can help reduce unplanned downtime is the predictive model that was developed for certain Magnetic Resonance Imagers (MRIs).

Problems had been reported with unplanned downtime by a number of hospitals using the MRIs manufactured by one particular company.

In response to these complaints, the manufacturer in collaboration with these hospitals, collected downtime data for a three-year period for 100 of the MRIs reporting problems.

Using this historical downtime data and machine learning software to identify patterns leading to reported equipment failure, the manufacturer was able to develop a prescriptive model which would alert each hospital as to when specific types of preventive maintenance should be performed on each MRI.

By following this prescriptive model's recommended timing for preventive maintenance, unplanned downtime for the MRIs at these hospitals was reduced by over 16%;[163] reducing and helping "prevent" unnecessary downtime, delays, and frustration for patients, staff and physicians.

5.5   Conduct Simulation Exercises

Repetition is important for "hardwiring" competence and proficiency in the performance of a given task or procedure.

Such "hardwiring" of behavior can help to "prevent" errors, mistakes, and/or potential harm to patients.

Not all tasks or procedures in healthcare, however, are performed on a regular or consistent basis.

163. Predictive maintenance of medical devices based on years of experience and advanced analytics, Case Studies, Hitachi
https://social-innovation.hitachi/en/case_studies/mri_predictive_maintenance/

Certain procedures or tasks in healthcare, however, may be performed infrequently or on an irregular basis, causing staff and clinicians difficulty in maintaining competence.

Use of simulation is one way of maintaining the staff and clinician competency needed to "prevent" mistakes or harm from occurring for such infrequently performed procedures.

By creating a specific scenario or situation that staff and clinicians must respond to (see appendix XIII), simulation helps "hardwire" the knowledge, skills, and protocols necessary to maintain the level of staff and clinician competence needed to "prevent" errors or mistakes from occurring which can cause injury or harm to patients.

A good example is fire in the OR.

Fires in the OR happen very infrequently (approximately 1 in every 90,000 cases).[164]

However, when a fire happens, it can have catastrophic consequences for the patient on the table if not handled quickly and appropriately by staff and surgeons; especially since almost all fires in the OR occur "in" or "on" the patient.[165]

Surgeons and staff generally have seconds to take the actions necessary to contain and extinguish a fire "in" or "on" a patient before the patient experiences serious harm.

When the cautery ignited the fumes from the alcohol-based prep that got trapped beneath the patient drapes, the surgeons and staff at one hospital knew exactly what to do...because they had simulated this

164. Kowalczyk, L. (2007). Fires during surgeries a bigger risk than thought. *Boston.com* November 7, 2007 http://archive.boston.com/news/local/articles/2007/11/07/fires_during_surgeries_a_bigger_risk_than_thought/

165. The Patient is on Fire! A Surgical Fires Primer, ECRI Institute, Guidance [Jan 1992;21(1):19-34] http://www.mdsr.ecri.org/summary/detail.aspx?doc_id=8197

exact scenario.

As a result, staff and physicians had the confidence and knowledge to quickly extinguish the fire "preventing" serious harm to the patient. [166]

Use of simulation is therefore one way of maintaining the staff and clinician competency needed to "prevent" mistakes or harm from occurring for infrequently performed activities and/or procedures.

166. Based on unpublished incident which occurred in a community hospital operating room.

CHAPTER 6
Leading Change

6.1   Knowledge is not Enough

Knowledge of how to assess, diagnose, treat, and prevent disease is important in the care of patients.

But knowledge of these areas is not enough.

To successfully manage the health of a patient takes more.

An understanding of the patient and how to influence the changes in attitude and behavior needed to ensure compliance with the recommended treatment plan is also required.

Prescribing a diabetic patient insulin and instructing them to manage their diet will not be of any help in controlling their blood sugar if the patient fails to check their insulin levels, administer insulin when needed, and make the dietary changes necessary.

The same goes for implementation of the principles of lean six sigma.

Knowledge of how to assess, diagnose, treat, and prevent "waste" and variation is not enough.

An understanding of how to successfully influence staff and clinician attitudes and behavior is also necessary to implement and sustain major organizational change; especially since an estimated one-third to two-thirds of all major change efforts fail.[167]

Some of the actions that can be taken to influence clinician and staff attitudes and behavior to successfully facilitate required changes include:

- Leveraging the organization's culture

- Creating an urgency for change

- Getting staff and physician buy-in

- Effectively managing staff and physician emotions

- Monitoring compliance, performance, and outcomes

- Providing frequent feedback and encouragement

6.2   Leveraging Organizational Culture

The culture of a department or organization exerts a strong influence over the attitudes and behaviors of individuals that work within that organization.

The culture of each department or organization is unique; stemming from the "shared" values and norms of the people that work within that department or organization.

Norms, which form the psychological foundation of a culture, have been shown to be even more powerful in the shaping of employee behavior

---

167. Gilley et al. (2009). Organizational Change: Motivation, Communication and Leadership Effectiveness. *Performance Improvement Quarterly* 21(4) pp 75-94, 2009
http://cstl-hcb.semo.edu/hmcmillan/Pubs/Gilley_Gilley_McMillan_2009.pdf

than either monetary rewards or physical work environment and demands. [168]

Leveraging these values and norms can therefore be instrumental in effecting successful change within a department or organization.

A good example of how an organization's culture can be leveraged to facilitate change was the *Proactive Office Encounter* (POE) initiative undertaken by a large multi-specialty group practice.

To improve the health of its managed care members, the group launched an organization wide *in-reach* initiative to identify preventive care gaps (i.e., need for mammogram screening, colorectal screening, out of control diabetic sugar, etc.) and provide the care and/or services needed to address any identified gaps.

Resistance from staff and clinicians was anticipated as they would be expected to inform patients of each care gap during every primary or specialty care visit and address them; creating "more" work for both staff and clinicians.

Since many people that pursue a career in healthcare are motivated by wanting to help people, this "shared" value was leveraged to help generate staff and clinician buy-in for the initiative.

By leveraging this shared value and the organization's culture of "preventive" medicine, the organization was able to overcome the resistance that did occur and successfully implement the *Proactive Office Encounter* initiative.

As a result of this initiative, coupled with a patient outreach program,

168. Chatman, J. & Cha, S. (2001). Leading by Leveraging Culture. December 11, 2001
http://www.hbs.edu/faculty/Publication%20Files/02-088_5a72f8e4-9c95-4a78-868c-c75c5c522746.pdf

patients with their blood pressure under control increased 44%, patients being screened for colon cancer increased 39%, patients with their cholesterol under control increased 35% and patients with HgA1C under control increased 15%.[169]

By providing patients with timely and appropriate preventive care, the *Proactive Office Encounter* along with the patient outreach program are expected to help save the lives of up to ten thousand patients per decade;[170] demonstrating the importance of proactive care and the power of leveraging an organization's culture to bring about change.

6.3   Creating an Urgency for Change

People exhibit a natural complacency if not outright resistance towards change.

These behaviors generally stem from people's comfort with the status quo and discomfort/reluctance to deviate from what they are already familiar with.[171]

People may feel more compelled to make changes, despite these psychological barriers, when they feel there is a sense of urgency or an

169. Lindsay, G. (2014). Transforming Care Delivery – Complete Care at Kaiser Permanente Southern California. *Open Forum*, Harvard Business School Digital Initiative Sep 4, 2014
https://www.hbs.edu/openforum/openforum.hbs.org/goto/challenge/hbs-hms-health-acceleration-challenge/transforming-care-delivery-complete-care-at-kaiser-permanente-southern-california.html

170. Fasano, P. (2013). Transforming Health Care.: The Financial Impact of Technology, Electronic Tools, and Data Mining. John Wiley and Sons 2013
https://books.google.com/books?id=Lx4i2brzh4IC&pg=PT104&lpg=PT104&dq=proactive+office+encounter+%2B+lives+saved&source=bl&ots=SOL7BvwSs&sig=ACfU3U1nGxaBgl7gfKRvQ0pvCjnCPukvvQ&hl=en&sa=X&ved=2ahUKEwim3qTAneDAhVGiVQKHaIXCXw4ChDoATAAegQICRAB#v=onepage&q=proactive%20office%20encounter%20%2B%20lives%20saved&f=false

171. Bolognese, A. (2018). Employee Resistance to Organizational Change
https://www.newfoundations.com/OrgTheory/Bolognese721.html

overwhelming need for change.[172]

Sometimes the urgency for change can result from an actual crisis that demands immediate action.

A good example of such a crisis is the occurrence of a never event in a hospital OR.

Surgeons and staff at one hospital were horrified when a never event, a wrong side surgery, occurred in their operating room.

This never event energized surgeons and staff to "want" to take action to prevent the occurrence of another such unacceptable incident; facilitating implementation of a number of major changes.

These changes included implementation of key elements of highly reliable surgical teams.

These elements which are designed to improve communication between members of the surgical team included:

- Flattening of the hierarchy (i.e., all members of surgical team use first names only)

- Conducting surgical briefings prior to the start of surgery

- Pausing and confirming critical information before incision

- Conducting a debriefing following surgery

- Standardizing the language team members use (i.e., use of SBAR) when communicating "critical" information

172. The Psychology of Urgency: 9 Ways to Drive Urgency, Content Partner, *Smart Insights*, June 26, 2018
https://www.smartinsights.com/digital-marketing-strategy/psychology-urgency-9-ways-drive-conversions/

By successfully "energizing" the surgeons and staff to adopt these procedural and behavioral changes, the OR achieved one of the highest safety ratings in the country on a safety measurement tool called the Safety Attitude Questionnaire (SAQ)[173] in addition to having one of the lowest incidences of never events nationally.[174]

An actual crisis such as this, however, is not always needed to create the sense of urgency or motivation needed to facilitate change.

A sense of urgency and need for change can also result from:

- Serious consequences of complacency or continuing to do what is being done

- Perceived benefit gained by staff or clinicians from making the change now

- Enthusiasm created by aspiration or achieving a shared vision

- Fear of personal loss

A good example is one medical group's effort to improve its patient satisfaction scores for staff service.

The Pacific Business Group on Health (PBGH) is a consortium of businesses that regularly conducts and publishes statistics on its members' satisfaction with the quality of health services received from the different medical groups that its members use.

Medical groups are rated on a number of satisfaction measures

---

173. Communication, collaboration, commitment are cornerstones of high reliability healthcare, *OR Manager*, volume 31 #3, March 2015

174. OR Excellence Awards, *Outpatient Surgery Magazine*, September 2009

including quality of care, patient's overall care experience, and the cost of care; with ratings of poor, fair, good, very good, and excellent.

One of the measures under overall patient care experience is staff helpfulness which evaluates the courteousness, helpfulness, and attentiveness of the medical group's employees.

Eighty-four percent (84%) of the medical groups in one of the geographic areas defined by PBGH received ratings during the previous year of "good" (2 stars) or less on the staff helpfulness measure.[175]

Dissatisfied with their poor results, one of the medical groups turned to internal satisfaction data to try to understand why they only rated "good" on this survey and work to improve patient perceptions of the service received from their staff.

Looking at internal satisfaction scores collected by individual employee for courtesy, helpfulness, and attentiveness; they determined that only 30% of their staff consistently received patient ratings of 90% or greater *highly satisfied* on all three measures of service.[176]

Wanting to improve perceptions, leadership set out to increase the percent of staff scoring 90% *highly satisfied* or higher on all three of these service measures.

To create a sense of urgency, leadership shared the PBGH ratings with the staff; emphasizing the impact it could have on membership...and the potential for organizational growth, jobs, and viability.

175. PBGH commercial rating for 28 medical groups for 2014-15 in the geographic area called Los Angeles West which reflected survey responses for the year 2013.
https://reportcard.opa.ca.gov/rc2015/medicalgrouptopic.aspx?Category=PAS&Topic=HelpfulOfficeStaff&County=LOS_ANGELES_WEST

176. Based on results of unpublished study of patient satisfaction ratings of individual clerical and nursing staff service performance pre training which reflected internal survey responses from 2013 outpatient visits.

This was then followed by intensive training which included role playing, videotaping, and feedback, to build and hardwire the individual service skills needed by each employee.

Individual service scores were then shared regularly with each employee; allowing them to track their progress and improvement against the rest of the employees in the department.

Sharing of this information added a sense of competitiveness and further urgency for each employee to make the changes in attitude and behavior needed to improve both individual and collective performance.

After taking these actions, the number of individual staff receiving ratings of 90% or greater *highly satisfied* on all three service measures jumped by 40 percentage points,[177] followed by improved ratings on the PBGH survey (see graph on next page); with the medical group receiving an "excellent" rating four stars) for staff helpfulness.[178]

Whether stemming from compelling information/feedback or an actual crisis, creating a sense of urgency can help motivate staff and/or physicians to make the changes in behavior and attitude needed to improve performance.

177. Based on results of unpublished study of patient satisfaction ratings of individual clerical and nursing staff service performance pre training which reflected internal survey responses from 2014 outpatient visits.

178. PBGH commercial rating for 32 medical groups for 2015-16 in the geographic area called Los Angeles West which reflected survey responses for the year 2014.
https://reportcard.opa.ca.gov/rc2016/medicalgrouptopic.aspx?Category=PAS&Topic=HelpfulOfficeStaff&County=LOS_ANGELES_WEST

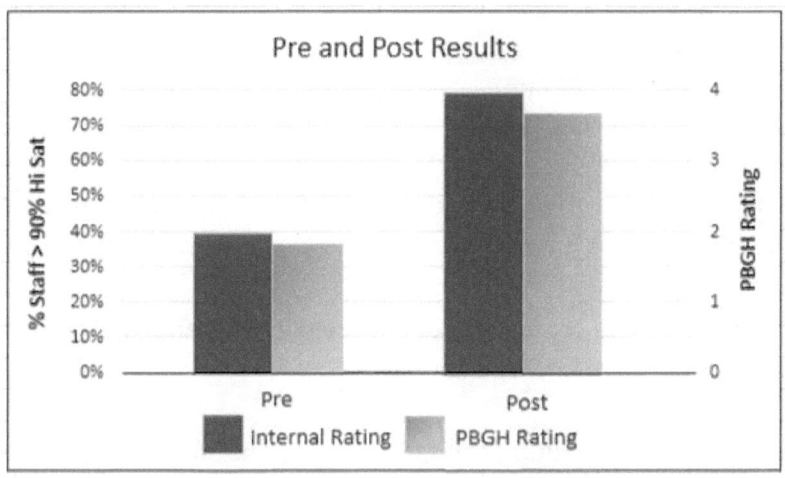

6.4 Managing Emotional Aspects of Change

Dying patients experience a number of emotions as they cope with the reality of their mortality and future.

The emotions and sequence they experience them in has been broken down into a series of stages called the Kubler Ross stages of loss.[179]

The Kubler Ross model identifies five (5) emotional stages a dying patient goes through.

These five stages and the sequence in which they occur are:

- Denial

- Anger

- Bargaining

179. Tyrrell et al. (2020). Stages of Dying. NCBI Bookshelf, Feb 19, 2020
https://www.ncbi.nlm.nih.gov/books/NBK507885/

- Depression

- Acceptance

Staff and physicians going through organizational changes experience similar stages of loss during the change process (see diagram below).

How these staff and clinician emotions are handled can significantly impact the success of any change effort.

A good example is the implementation of an electronic medical record (EMR) system.

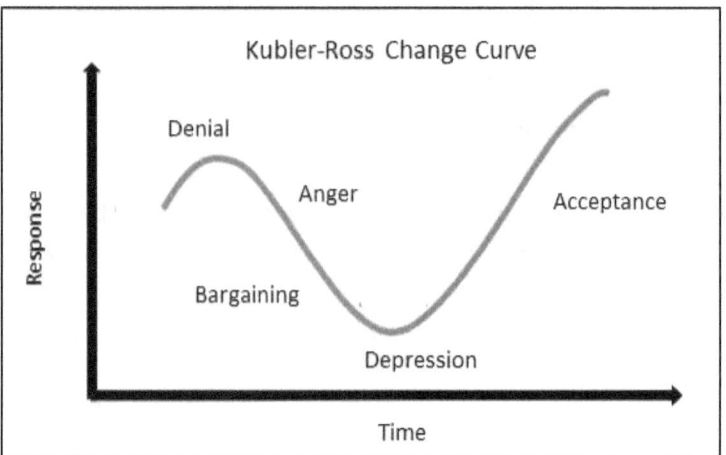

The paper charts were to be replaced by an electronic medical record system (EMR) at one large multi hospital system.

Following announcement of this decision, many of the staff and physicians throughout the organization were in denial; confident that the organization really wouldn't implement such a system because of the complexity and expense involved.

Denial was replaced by anger once physicians and staff realized that implementation of an EMR was inevitable.

Their anger centered around the loss of the paper record that they were comfortable using, the need to take time away from patient care to learn how to use the new system, and the need to acquire or enhance not only their typing skills but their typing speed.

As their anger gradually dissipated, staff and physicians began bargaining about various aspects of the implementation.

They tried to bargain about the timing and length of the roll out, the number of patients they could see while learning how to use the new system, and the length of time paper charts would continue to be provided following roll out of the new system.

Bargaining turned to depression as many of the staff and physicians struggled to learn the new system and became frustrated with the length of time it initially was taking them to enter notes, orders, and other key information into the system.

As staff and physicians became more proficient in the use of the system, their depression turned to acceptance; and eventually staff and physicians wondered how they were ever able to work with just paper charts rather than an electronic medical record.

Successful change management depends on helping staff and physicians progress through each of the five (5) different stages of grief and loss during the change process as quickly and painlessly as possible.

This can be accomplished by being visible and accessible to staff and physicians and taking the following actions to help physicians and staff navigate through each of the five (5) different stages of grief/loss:

- **EXPLAIN** to staff and physicians what changes are planned, why the changes are being made, and how they and their patients will benefit

- **PREPARE** staff and physicians for the types of emotional responses they may experience during the upcoming change *(i.e., During the implementation process you may experience the following five (5) emotional responses to the changes being made)*

- **ACKNOWLEDGE** staff and physician feelings at each stage of the grief/loss cycle *(i.e., I understand that you're angry that you are having to take time away from patient care to learn how to use the system)*

- **NORMALIZE** staff and physician feelings at each stage of the grief/loss cycle *(i.e., It is normal to feel such emotions during the change process)*

- **REFRAME** staff and physician perspectives towards the change *(i.e., Imagine how happy you'll feel when you won't have to deal with lost charts or illegible notes)*

By recognizing the five (5) stages of grief/loss during the change process and what actions to take if observed, many of the problems commonly encountered when implementing change can be minimized, if not totally avoided.

6.5   Involvement and Buy In

Most successful change initiatives have one thing in common; they have the support of staff and physicians.

Getting the support from staff and physicians often requires more than just having a clear explanation, understanding, and justification for the change.

It also requires staff and physician involvement; particularly in various aspects of planning and decision-making.[180]

Such involvement can range from having staff and physicians participate in actually making the decisions on "what" changes to make and "how" they should be implemented to merely getting staff and physician feedback and concerns about planned changes.

A good example is how one large multi-specialty group involved physicians in changes to the referral process.

In this organization, patient access to most specialists was by referral only.

Patients were therefore forced to be seen and evaluated by their primary care physician before being seen by a specialist.

Patients complained that this practice was wasteful and overly restrictive; causing unnecessary delays in treatment, unnecessary visits to primary care doctors, and was more costly as a result of having to pay multiple copays.

Specialists, however, were resistant to allowing patients to self-refer as they were concerned that they would be inundated with patients having problems that could easily be treated by the patients' primary care physicians.

To overcome this resistance and instill a sense of physician ownership in the move towards patient self-referral, several key physicians from each specialty department were asked to participate in helping make the decision as to "which" medical problems for their specialty would be appropriate for self-referral.

180. Nielsen, K. & Randall, R. (2012). The importance of employee participation and perceptions of changes in procedures in a teamworking environment. *Work Stress*. 2012 Apr; 26(2): 91–111.
https://www.ncbi.nlm.nih.gov/pmc/articles/PMC3379743/

After determining which medical problems would be appropriate for self-referral, the physicians then helped decide "what" screening criteria the appointment clerks would use to identify patients that could be directly booked into their department without a referral.

After successfully piloting the self-referral criteria with a few physicians in each department, the program was then rolled out for all physicians.

Following implementation, self-referrals ended up accounting for approximately 20 percent of all new visits to specialty departments;[181] significantly improving patient satisfaction with access to specialists.

And contrary to physician concerns, there was no significant increase in the total volume of new patient visits to each specialty department;[181] facilitating further expansion of the self-referral criteria for a number of the specialty departments within the medical group and demonstrating the importance of staff and physician involvement and buy in in the change process.

6.6   Leading the Way

What leadership does is more important than what leadership says.

This is particularly true during the change process where staff and physicians may question or not be fully committed to the changes being implemented.

Leadership must not only encourage and promote the change; leadership must "lead" the way...and role model the changes being implemented.

Otherwise staff and physicians will question leadership's commitment ... and be resistant, if not outright noncompliant, with the changes

181. Results of unpublished study from a multi-specialty clinic.

needed.

A good example of how leadership actions can affect staff and physician behavior was the implementation of leadership rounding at one medical center.

Rounding is the management practice of physically visiting a work area to observe what is happening in that work environment and solicit input and information from staff and patients about the quality, safety, and opportunities for improvement of the care and services provided.

Senior leadership at this medical center decided it needed to formalize the rounding process since it was felt that managers spent too much time in their offices and not enough time in their departments.

The expectation was that every manager in the medical center, including senior leaders, would make rounds at least twice per day; with reporting of rounds monthly, along with findings, to the Director of Service.

The number of rounds made per month by each manager were tracked and compiled by the Director of Service into a monthly report that was then distributed to all managers (including senior leaders).

After several months, the rate of compliance with the daily rounding goals plateaued at less than 30%; with over 70% of managers, including the senior leaders, not complying with the expectations that had been set.

The failure of senior leaders to set, but not role model, the expected behaviors resulted in this change initiative just petering out over time; reinforcing why what leadership *does* is as important, if not more important, than what leadership *says*.

6.7   Monitoring Compliance

One of the realities of implementing change is that the roll out and change process often do not go as planned.

Unanticipated issues or problems may occur which can adversely impact the success of the rollout or the effectiveness of the intended changes.

Such issues or problems can often be surfaced by monitoring the roll out process and, once identified, taking the steps needed to mitigate the problem.

The most common approaches employed for monitoring the change process include:

- **ROUNDING** on staff and clinicians to observe and verify that prescribed changes to policy, procedure, and practice have been incorporated into their daily workflow

- **TALKING** with staff and clinicians to identify what changes they have made, problems they may be encountering, and their perceived effectiveness of the changes

- **COLLECTING** key quality, service, or outcome data and tracking using Statistical Process Control (SPC) to determine the effectiveness or lack thereof of the changes made

A good example of how problems can be surfaced by monitoring key aspects of the change process is provided by the efforts of one medical group to improve the collection of copays at point of service.

Many of the patients being seen by physicians in this organization asked to be billed for services rather than pay by cash, check, or credit card at the point of service.

Since the amount of each copay was often nominal, the cost of actually processing, billing, and collecting these charges often exceeded the cost of the copay.

To increase the percent of copays collected at the point of service, staff were told to charge patients a nominal $5 processing fee if they chose to be billed rather than make their payment at the point of service.

While a reduction in the percent of patients choosing to be billed was expected, monitoring of the collection rate using an SPC control chart showed no statistically significant reduction in the number of patients who chose to be billed (see graph below).[182]

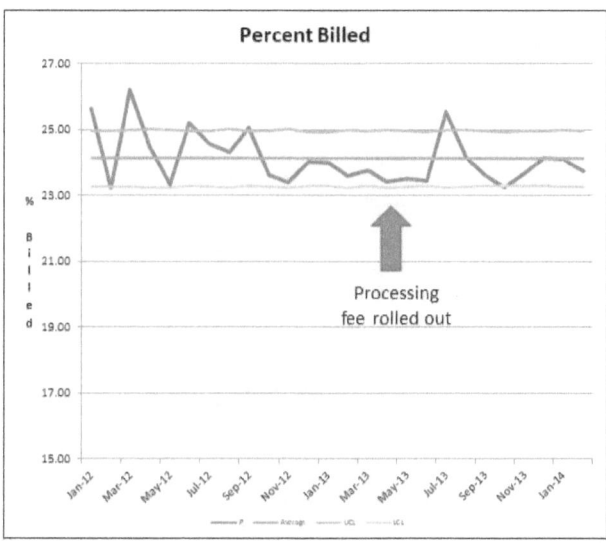

Talking to staff and conducting random observations showed that staff were slow in adopting and using this tactic; primarily because of the angry response they were getting from patients to the change in policy.

Working with staff from marketing, new messaging was developed to assist receptionists more successfully communicate the changes in

182. Based on results from unpublished study of billing and collection rates from one multi-specialty group clinic.

billing policy to patients.

This messaging was then reinforced with the staff through role playing, additional training directed towards dealing with angry patients, and the posting of appropriate signage at patient check in locations.

Staff confidence and comfort increased following roll out of these initiatives; leading to improved staff communication with patients and a statistically significant drop in the number of copays being billed rather than collected at the point of service (see below).[183]

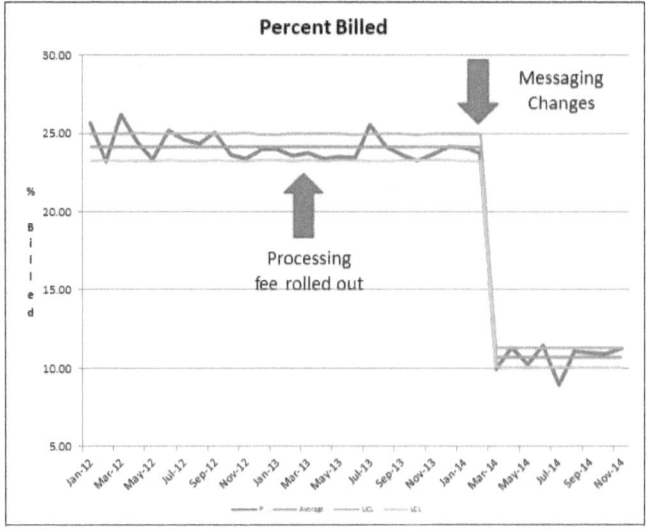

By identifying and monitoring key aspects of both conformance and performance during the implementation process (as illustrated in this case), issues and problems can be more quickly surfaced, evaluated, and resolved.

183. Based on results from unpublished study of billing and collection rates from one multi-specialty group clinic.

6.8   Feedback and Encouragement

Feedback and encouragement to staff and physicians during the change process is crucial for successful implementation of change.

Feedback lets staff and physicians know what is going well... and what isn't; reinforcing desired behaviors while encouraging changes in unwanted or unacceptable behaviors.

A good example of the importance of feedback and encouragement in the change process is the initiative undertaken at one hospital to start its operating rooms on time.

The Operating Room is typically the most expensive department in a hospital.

Delays in the start of surgery are not only extremely costly and disruptive to an operating room's schedule, but also cause frustration for patients, staff, and surgeons.

At one hospital, only 50% of the first cases of the day were found to start by 7:30 A.M. or "on time".[184]

A number of factors were found to contribute to the delay in starting the first case of the day on time including missing labs, incomplete documentation, and missing instrument trays and equipment.

Late surgeon arrival, however, was the most significant problem; accounting for over 70% of all cases that did not start "on time".[184]

Surgeons were therefore reminded that they needed to be in the preop area by 7:15 A.M. to mark their first patient of the day.

184. Based on results from unpublished study of on time starts in the operating room at a mid-sized hospital.

Their arrival times were then tracked; and feedback/encouragement provided to them about their individual arrival time history.

Those surgeons that consistently arrived on time received praise and encouragement while those surgeons that were consistently late were reminded about the need for punctuality and informed that their morning block time privileges would be rescinded in the absence of improvement.

Surgeon punctuality improved in response to the individual feedback and encouragement provided; increasing the percent of "on time" starts to 95 percent of all first cases.[184]

Similar results were reported in another hospital where similar actions were taken which resulted in a 50-percentage point increase in "on time" starts; demonstrating the importance of feedback and encouragement in changing behaviors during the change management process.[185]

6.9   Take ACTION

Finally, leading change requires **ACTION !**

Without taking action, nothing gets done.

Having read this book and learned:

1.   What "*Muda*" or "waste" is

2.   How "waste" can be identified

185. Darwish et al. (2016). Improving operating room start times in a community teaching hospital. *Journal of Hospital Administration* 2016, Vol. 5, No. 3
http://www.sciedu.ca/journal/index.php/jha/article/view/8325/5451

3. How "waste" affects the costs and quality of healthcare

4. How the cause(s) of "waste" can be determined

5. What actions can be taken to reduce or eliminate "waste" to reduce costs and/or improve quality, access, or service

6. What actions can be taken to prevent "waste"

7. How the changes and improvements you make can be sustained

it is now time for **YOU** to take **ACTION** and **LEAD** the way by applying the knowledge and skills you have acquired to identify and eliminate waste within your organization in order to trim away the fat and improve the access, quality, and service you and your staff provide to your organization's patients and customers.

APPENDICES

APPENDIX I

The Six Domains of Quality

The six domains of quality[186] include:

1. **SAFE** and avoiding harm to patients from the care that is intended to help them

2. **EFFECTIVE** and providing services based on scientific knowledge and evidence to those who can benefit while refraining from providing services to those not likely to benefit

3. **PATIENT-CENTERED** and providing care that is respectful of and responsive to individual patient preferences, needs, and values and ensuring that patient values guide all clinical decisions

4. **TIMELY** and reducing waits and sometimes harmful delays for both those who receive and those who give care

5. **EFFICIENT** and avoiding waste, including waste of equipment, supplies, ideas, and energy

6. **EQUITABLE** and providing care that does not vary in quality because of personal characteristics such as gender, ethnicity, geographic location, and socioeconomic status

186. Six Domains of Healthcare Quality, Agency for Healthcare Research and Quality, November 2018
https://www.ahrq.gov/talkingquality/measures/six-domains.html

APPENDIX II

Differences Between Six Sigma and Lean

The differences between Six Sigma and Lean include:

SIX SIGMA	LEAN
Reduces variation	Removes waste
Improves quality	Increases speed
Reduces variation at each remaining step	Removes non value-added process steps
Optimizes remaining process steps	Fixes connections between process steps
Uses DMAIC improvement model	Uses PDCA or PDSA improvement model

The SIX SIGMA IMPROVEMENT MODEL consists of the following five (5) steps versus the PDSA or PDCA process typically used in Lean:

DEFINE	MEASURE	ANALYZE	IMPROVE	CONTROL
• What is the problem? • What is the impact of problem? • What is the goal or objective? • How is success measured?	• What data should be collected? • How should data be collected? • Who will collect data? • Collect data	• How should data be organized? • What does data mean? • How does data compare to goals?	• What opportunities are available? • What actions should be taken? • Take action	• Monitor • How can improvements be sustained?

APPENDIX III

Common Flowchart Symbols

The most commonly used symbols for constructing a flowchart include the following:

Process	▭	Storage	▽	Document	▭	Manual Input	▱
Transport	⇒	Connector	○	Database	⬭	Display	⬠
Decision	◇	Preparation	⬡	Sort	◈	Manual Operation	⏢
Delay	D	Data	▱	Collate	⋈	Terminator	⬭

APPENDIX IV

<u>Translating Random Numbers to Times</u>

Random numbers from a random numbers table are translated into the times a sample is to be taken by following the steps below:

1. An 8-hour shift equals 480 minutes

2. Start with any random number in the table on the next page

3.   For this example, start with the first random number which is 63271 which would translate into minute 271

4. Proceed down the table to the next number which is 88547 which would translate into minute 47 since 547 exceeds the number of minutes in the shift

5. Keep moving down the table translating the numbers into minutes until an adequate number of observations have been identified to get the required sample size (see appendix V for instructions on how to calculate sample sizes)

RANDOM NUMBERS

63271	59986	71744	51102	15141	80714	58683	93108	13554	79945
88547	09896	95436	79115	08303	01041	20030	63754	08459	28364
55957	57243	83865	09911	19761	66535	40102	26646	60147	15702
46276	87453	44790	67122	45573	84358	21625	16999	13385	22782
55363	07449	34835	15290	76616	67191	12777	21861	68689	03263
69393	92785	49902	58447	42048	30378	87618	26933	40640	16281
13186	29431	88190	04588	38733	81290	89541	70290	40113	08243
17726	28652	56836	78351	47327	18518	92222	55201	27340	10493
36520	64465	05550	30157	82242	29520	69753	72602	23756	54935
81628	36100	39254	56835	37636	02421	98063	89641	64953	99337
84649	48968	75215	75498	49539	74240	03466	49292	36401	45525
63291	11618	12613	75055	43915	26488	41116	64531	56827	30825
70502	53225	03655	05915	37140	57051	48393	91322	25653	06543
06426	24771	59935	49801	11082	66762	94477	02494	88215	27191
20711	55609	29430	70165	45406	78484	31639	52009	18873	96927
41990	70538	77191	25860	55204	73417	83920	69468	74972	38712
72452	36618	76298	26678	89334	33938	95567	29380	75906	91807
37042	40318	57099	10528	09925	89773	41335	96244	29002	46453
53766	52875	15987	46962	67342	77592	57651	95508	80033	69828
90585	58955	53122	16025	84299	53310	67380	84249	25348	04332
32001	96293	37203	64516	51530	37069	40261	61374	05815	06714
62606	64324	46354	72157	67248	20135	49804	09226	64419	29457
10078	28073	85389	50324	14500	15562	64165	06125	71353	77669
91561	46145	24177	15294	10061	98124	75732	00815	83452	97355
13091	98112	53959	79607	52244	63303	10413	63839	74762	50289

APPENDIX V

Calculating Required Sample Sizes for Work Sampling

Required sample sizes for work sampling are calculated by taking the following steps:

1. Define the confidence level and margin of error desired for observations

2. Calculate the required sample size for observations using either the statistical method or the nomogram method described below:

STATISTICAL METHOD

1. Take a preliminary sample (note: a sample taken at random from a large population provides a good estimate of the distribution of the population)

2. Define the confidence level and margin of error desired for observations

3. Select the appropriate standard deviation from the table below for the confidence level desired

Confidence Level	Standard Deviation
80%	1.28
85%	1.44
90%	1.64
95%	1.96
98%	2.33
99%	2.58
99.9%	3.3

4. Use the following formula to calculate the sample size required

$$N = \frac{(Z^2)\,(P)\,(1-P)}{(S^2)}$$

where

N = sample size or observations required
S = desired relative accuracy
P = percentage occurrence of an activity
Z = standard deviation for desired confidence level
    (see table on previous page)

<u>EXAMPLE</u>

Assume that 100 observations were randomly performed as a preliminary study which showed that a machine was idle 25% of the time (p = 25).

Assume a confidence level of 95% is desired with a 5% margin of error (in other words, be confident that in 95% of cases the results obtained will be within ± 5% of the real value):

    S = 5% or 0.05
    P = 25% or 0.25
    Z = 1.96 for a 95% confidence level

$$N = \frac{(1.96^2)\,(0.25)\,(1-0.25)}{(0.05^2)} = 300 \text{ observations}$$

A sample of 300 observations would therefore be required to have a 95%

level of confidence that the results are within ± 5% of the real value (which in this case is the percent of time the machine was idle).

NOMOGRAM METHOD

Another way of determining the number of observations required is to use a nomogram.

A nomogram is a diagram which represents the relationship between three or more variable quantities by means of a number of scales.

These scales are arranged so that the value of one variable can be found by a simple geometric construction, for example, by drawing a straight line intersecting the other scales at the appropriate values (see nomogram on next page).

To use the nomogram

1. Take a preliminary sample

2. Identify the percentage occurrence (p) from the sample and mark it on the first scale

3. Identify the margin of error desired and mark it on the second scale

4. Draw a line through the two points to the third scale to find the number of observations required

The nomogram on the next page demonstrates how the number of observations required would be determined using the same assumptions made in the statistical method example (P = 25%, S = 5%, and confidence level = 95%).

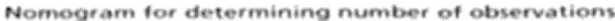

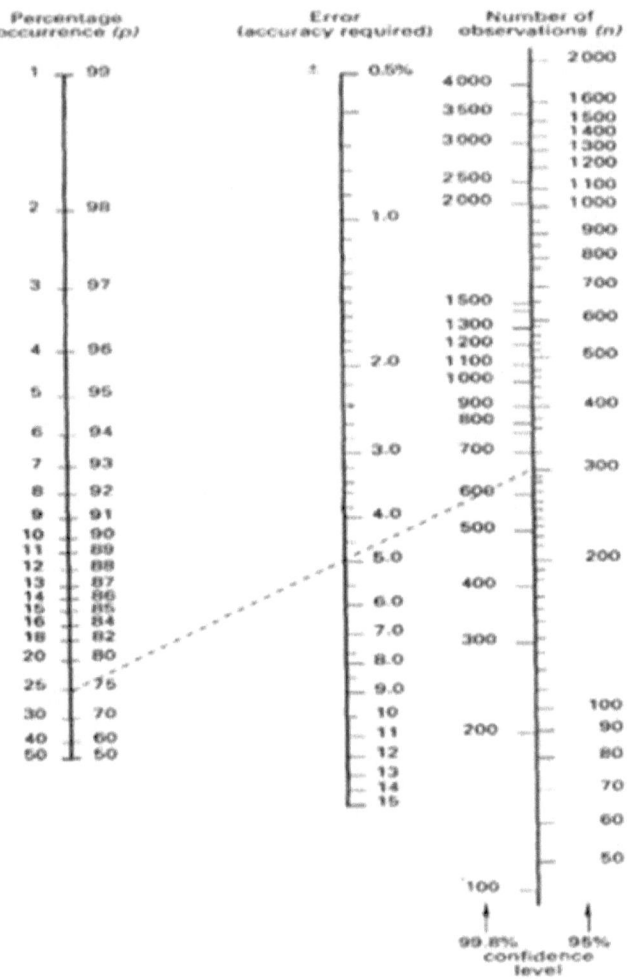

Nomogram for determining number of observations

Note: Sample sizes at the 90% and 99% confidence level, respectively, can be obtained by multiplying 0.70 and 1.75 with the number obtained for the 95% confidence level. [187]

187. Malhotra, R. & Indrayan, A. (2010). A simple nomogram for sample size for estimating sensitivity and specificity of medical tests. *Indian J Ophthalmol*. 2010 Nov-Dec; 58(6): 519–522

APPENDIX VI

Patient Satisfaction Data: Wait Time in MD Office

A survey[188] conducted of over 5000 patients of patient wait times for their doctor found that:

1. 55% of patients reported waiting over 15 minutes with 15% waiting 31 minutes or more

2. Although almost half the patients waited less than 15 minutes to see their md, 97% said they were frustrated by their wait times

3. More than 40% of patients reported they'd be willing to see another doctor in the practice if it meant a shorter wait time

REPORTED WAIT TIMES FOR MD

Wait time	Percent
< 15 min	45%
15-30 min	40%
31-60 min	9%
> 60 min	6%

WILLING TO SEE ANOTHER MD

Willingness	Percent
Willing to see another md	41%
Not willing to see another md	59%

188. Software Advice
https://www.slideshare.net/SoftwareAdvice/the-cure-for-wait-time-woes-software-advice-industry-view

Another survey found that patient satisfaction with wait time to see their doctor had a significant impact on their overall visit satisfaction and declined precipitously after even a relatively short wait for their doctor.[189]

Star Rating	Average Wait Time
5	12 min, 56 sec
4	18 min, 19 sec
3	21 min, 40 sec
2	26 min, 11 sec
1	33 min, 1 sec

Another survey found the following relationship between wait time and overall visit satisfaction.[190]

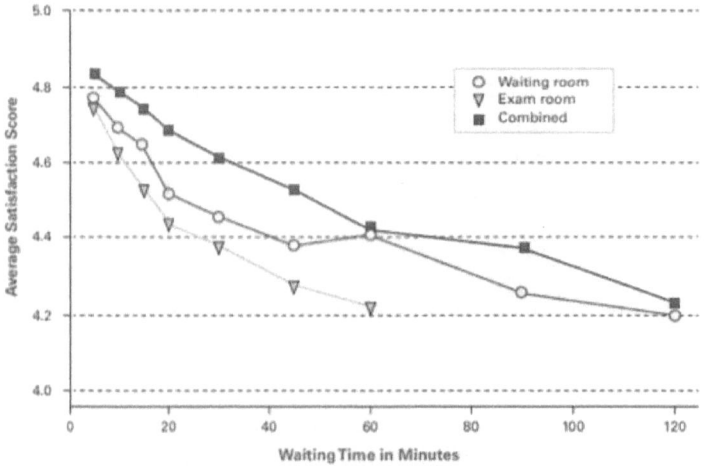

189. Report: Patient Satisfaction Tanks After 20-Minute Doctor Wait Time, HITC Staff, 3/24/16
https://hitconsultant.net/2016/03/24/report-patient-satisfaction-tanks-20-minute-doctor-wait-time/

190. Bleustein et al. (2014). Wait Times, Patient Satisfaction Scores, and the Perception of Care, *The American Journal of Managed Care*, Vol 20 No 5, 2014: 393 - 400

APPENDIX VII

Patient Satisfaction Data: Appointment Access

Timely access to care is 1 of the 6 dimensions of health care quality identified by the Institute of Medicine's report, *Crossing the Quality Chasm*.[191]

One study found that only 44% of adults were always able to get routine care as soon as desired, while 57% of adults were always able to get illness or injury care as soon as desired.[191]

Another study found that patients expected to be seen sooner than physicians thought necessary for most common chronic medical conditions. However, patients and physicians were generally found to be in agreement about timeliness for acute problems.[191]

This study also found that patients had a greater perception of urgency than physicians did especially related to access for chronic conditions.[191]

Another study found the following relationship between patient satisfaction for new and established patients and days wait to be seen (see graph on next page).[192]

Another study found the following relationship between patient satisfaction for patients with and without a primary care provider (PCP),

191. Barry et al. (2006). Patient and Physician Perceptions of Timely Access to Care, *J Gen Intern Med*. 2006 Feb; 21(2): 130–133.
https://www.ncbi.nlm.nih.gov/pmc/articles/PMC1484658/#!po=1.00000

192. Harte, B. & Hixson, E. Leveraging the Relationship Between Days Wait to Appointment and Outpatient Satisfaction Scores to Improve Retention Rates, Reimbursement, and Reporting Metrics, Cleveland Clinic.
https://na.eventscloud.com/file_uploads/00ac01b2f12f9f04c0f2205c65f6a8e3_HarteHixson.pdf

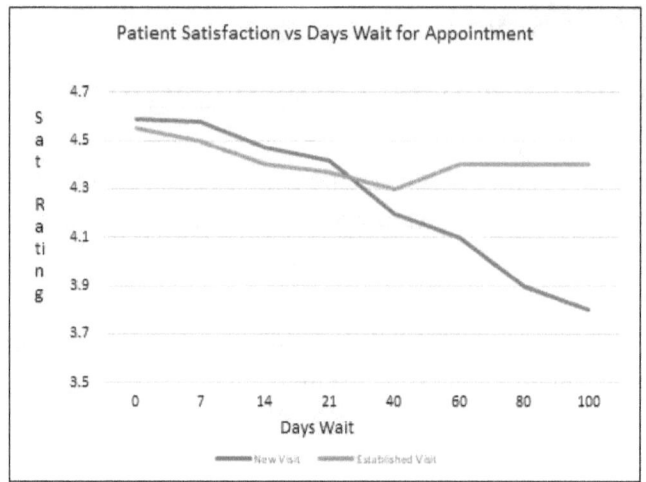

days wait to be seen, and whether or not they saw their own PCP (see graph below).[193]

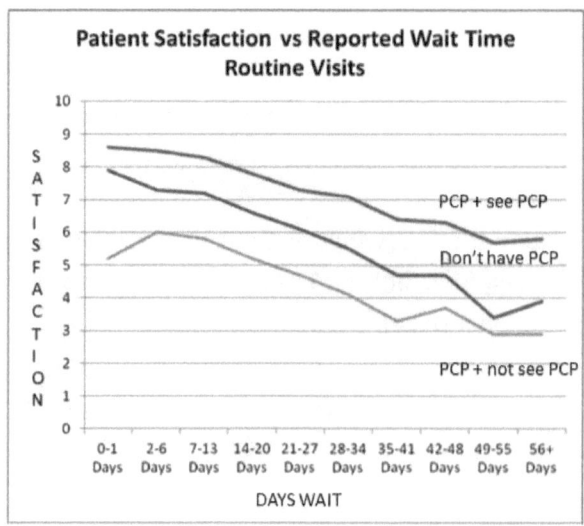

193. Results of an unpublished analysis of the relationship between patient satisfaction and wait time for appointments.

APPENDIX VIII

Single Minute Exchange Die (SMED)

The concept of Single Minute Die Exchange is derived from the manufacturing industry.

In healthcare the SMED equivalent is called set-up, clean-up, or turnover time.

SMED is typically broken down into three stages. Each stage has specific tasks and objectives and all are inter-related and work together. Those steps are outlined below:

Step 1 – Separate internal and external setup

Step 2 – Convert internal setup to external setup

Step 3 – Streamline internal and external elements

The impact of these actions on changeover or turnover time are Illustrated below:

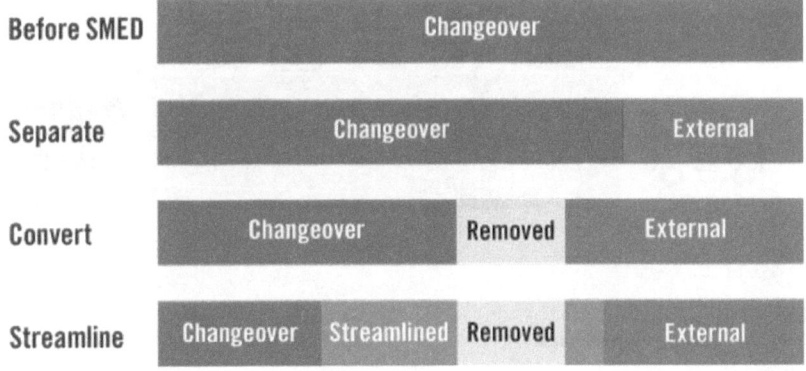

APPENDIX IX

One Piece Flow

The concept of one-piece flow comes from the manufacturing industry.

The underlying principle of one-piece flow is commonly referred to as **"make one, move one"** (see below).

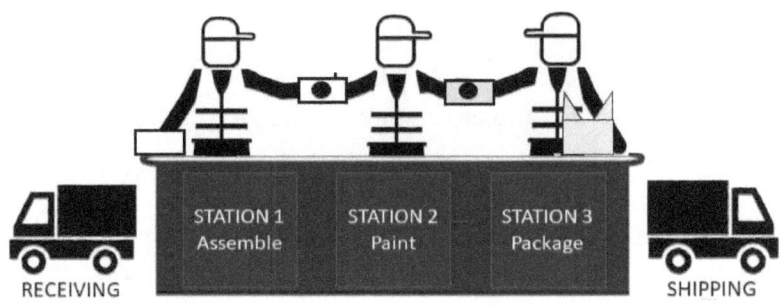

This is in contrast to mass production which is **"make many before moving any"** (see below).

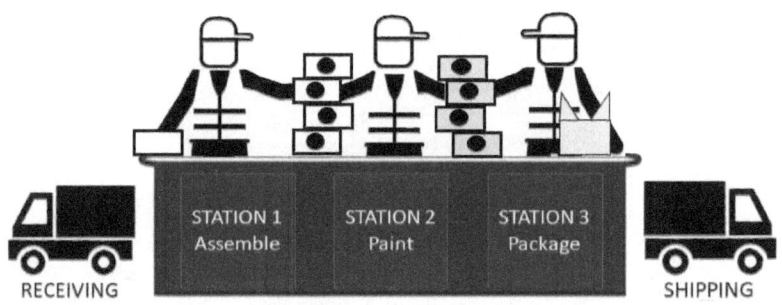

Picture Images adapted from::

Lean Enterprise Institute
https://www.lean.org/lexicon/continuous-flow

In manufacturing, to be a good candidate for one-piece flow, a process should meet the following conditions[194]:

1. The process must be able to consistently produce a quality product that meets established standards

2. *Process times must be repeatable and have little variation from cycle to cycle*

3. Equipment, if required, must be available to run when needed

4. Processes must be able to be scaled to takt time, or the rate of customer demand (i.e., if takt time is 10 minutes, processes should be able to scaled to run at one unit every 10 minutes)

The steps that are normally taken to implement one-piece flow in industry include[194]:

Step 1   Determine which products or product families will be included in the cells, and determine the type of cell (i.e. product-focused or mixed model)

(Note: A cell is the logical grouping or physical arrangement of equipment, workers, materials and supplies used to produce a product/service or mix of products/services in one physical location or close proximity)

Step 2   Calculate the takt time for the set of products/services that will go into the cell

Step 3   Determine the work elements and time required for making one piece or serving one customer

Step 4   Determine if the equipment or process to be used within the cell can meet takt time considering changeover times, load and unload times, and downtime

194. Dolcemascolo, D. Achieving one-piece flow. ReliablePlant
https://www.reliableplant.com/Read/14703/one-piece-flow

Step 5   Create a lean layout using the principles of 5S and eliminate items that are not needed and locate all items/equipment/materials/workers that are needed at their points of use in the proper sequence

Step 6   Balance the cell, determine the number of workers required, split the work between operators, create standardized work for each operator within the cell

Flow in healthcare may also be defined by some as the "8 flows"[195] which is broken down as the FLOW of:

- Patients
- Family
- Clinicians
- Medications
- Supplies
- Equipment
- Information
- Processes

Optimizing patient flow and the patient care experience according to others requires the presence of all (or most of) the following 6 rights[196]:

1. The right resources

2. To the right patient

3. In the right environment

4. For the right reasons

5. With the right team

6. At the right time, *everytime*

195. The Flows of Medicine, Virginia Mason Institute, 7/31/17
https://www.virginiamasoninstitute.org/the-flows-of-medicine-2/

196. Jensen, K. & Mayer, T. (2009). Hardwiring Flow: Systems and Processes for Seamless Patient Care, Fire Starter Publishing, 2009, page 20

APPENDIX X

Calculating the Reserve Stock Required

The calculation for the amount of inventory to be kept in the reserve stock bin is:

(Daily usage rate × Lead time) + <u>Safety stock</u> = Reserve bin quantity

EXAMPLE

Assumptions:

- A pharmacy uses 500 bottles/week of a brand name drug (5-day week)
- Lead time is three (3) days from reorder to receipt of order
- Usage can vary by as much as 25% from the average daily usage

Steps:

1. Calculate the daily usage rate

   500 bottles/5 days = 100 bottles/day

2. Calculate the number of bottles required to cover the expected usage during the 3-day lead time

   100 bottles/day x 3 days = 300 bottles

3. Calculate the maximum variation from average usage

   25% x 100 bottles/day x 3-day lead time = 75 bottles

4. Calculate the total reserve stock required

   300 average bottles + 75 bottles = 375 bottles
   (from Step 2)   (from Step 3)

APPENDIX XI

<u>Calculating Cycle Time</u>

Cycle time is the time starting when a task or operation begins to the point of time when the task or operation ends.

Cycle time can be calculated by observation, time study, estimation, or extrapolation.

The simplest (but less precise) method for calculating cycle time is to do an estimation of the time required to produce or service one unit, customer, or order.

To estimate the cycle time, take the total production or service hours and divide by the number of units made or serviced during that time.

> <u>EXAMPLE</u>
>
> The receptionist at a medical office building checks in an average of 48 patients in a half day (4 hours).[197]
>
> The estimated cycle time would be 5 minutes.
>
> Cycle Time = $\dfrac{\text{4 hours x (60 minutes/hour)}}{\text{48 patients}}$ = 5 minutes/patient

A more precise way to calculate the cycle time for this process, however, would be to use observation or time study.

To calculate cycle time using observation or time study:

197. Carroll, J. (2015). Patient Check-In: One of the most important processes in improving your bottom line. *Advantage Health Care Consulting* April 17, 2015
https://www.advadm.com/patient-check-in-one-of-the-most-important-processes-in-improving-your-bottom-line/

LEAN HEALTHCARE

1. Determine the bounds for the process to be measured (i.e. beginning point and end point)

2. Determine the appropriate sample size to collect

3. Observe and record a sample of cycle times

4. Calculate the average cycle time for all observations

EXAMPLE

Steps:

1. Determine the bounds for the process to be measured

      Beginning point: Greeting of patient
      End point: Patient given directions to waiting room/leaves reception desk

2. Determine the appropriate sample size

      See Appendix V

3. Observe and record the required sample of cycle times

| CYCLE TIME OBSERVATIONS ||
OBSERVATION	TIME (minutes)
1	4.5
2	5.0
3	4.5
4	4.5
5	6.1
6	4.5
7	4.0
8	5.0
9	5.5
10	4.5
Total	48.1

4. Calculate the average cycle time for all observations

CYCLE TIME OBSERVATIONS	
OBSERVATION	TIME (minutes)
1	4.5
2	5.0
3	4.5
4	4.5
5	6.1
6	4.5
7	4.0
8	5.0
9	5.5
10	4.5
Total	48.1
Mean	4.8
Median	4.5

Mean cycle time in this example is calculated to be 4.8 minutes and median cycle time is 4.5 minutes for a receptionist to check-in a patient

Cycle time can be used along with TAKT time to identify potential problems with FLOW.

Issues in production or service will occur when the cycle time is longer than the takt time (means machine or workers not able to meet demand).

APPENDIX XII

Impact of Poor Employees

According to one survey conducted of employees, low performing employees have a significant adverse effect on an organization.

These effects include:

- Lowering overall workplace morale (per 68% of respondents)

- Increasing the work burden on high performers (per 44% of respondents)

- Contributing to a lack of initiative and motivation, resulting in a work culture where mediocrity is accepted (per 54% of respondents)[198]

Low-performing workers don't just affect their peers; they also consume a large chunk of their manager's time.

Another survey revealed that some managers spend 17% of their time, the equivalent of nearly one day a week, managing poor performers.[198]

Another survey found that about 16% of the people in any job fall into the "superior" category, 16% in the "poor performer" category, and the remainder into the "average performer" category.[199]

A study out of Northwestern University found that sitting within 25 feet

198. Williams, T. Don't Let Low Performers Destroy Your Company. *The Economist*
https://execed.economist.com/blog/career-hacks/dont-let-low-performers-destroy-your-company

199. Poor Performing Employees Severely Impact Productivity, Robert Cameron and Associates, streetdirectory.com
https://www.streetdirectory.com/travel_guide/20418/corporate_matters/poor_performing_employees_severely_impact_productivity.html

of a high performer at work improved an employee's performance by 15 percent. But sitting within 25 feet of a low performer hurt their performance by 30 percent.[200]

According to another study, 47 percent of high performing employees are actively looking for other jobs, while only 18% of low performers are actively looking for jobs meaning that many organizations end up getting stuck with their poor performing employees and not retaining their high performing employees.[201]

200. Ranzetta, T. (2019). QoD: How much of a decline in performance (in percent) comes from sitting next to a low performer at work? *Next Gen Personal Finance* Mar 26, 2019
https://www.ngpf.org/blog/career/qod-how-much-of-a-decline-in-performance-in-percent-comes-from-sitting-next-to-a-low-performer-at-work/

201. Workplace poll finds high performers are ready to quit, ReliablePlant, Noria
https://www.reliableplant.com/Read/10393/workplace-poll-finds-high-performers-are-ready-to-quit-

APPENDIX XIII

Elements of a Simulation Scenario

There are several types of simulations that are commonly used to prepare staff and physicians for high risk or infrequently performed tasks or activities.

The most common types of simulations found in healthcare include:

1. **DRILLS** *which are structured exercises usually employed to test, practice, or reinforce a process or activity within a single entity (i.e., a department conducts a decontamination drill)*

2. **TABLETOP EXERCISES** *which involve a discussion or simulated response to a situation or incident which is played out in a conference room or informal setting to practice and assess the effectiveness of plans, policies, and/or procedures*

3. **FUNCTONAL OR FULL-SCALE SIMULATIONS** *which are interactive exercises simulating an actual emergency, disaster, or situation which requires the actual deployment and response of staff and/or equipment to the incident in order to practice, maintain, and improve the effectiveness of the response*

The basic steps required to prepare for a simulation may, depending on the type of simulation, require the following:

1. Determining areas of risk or training opportunities

2. Developing the simulation scenario, goals, and outcomes

3. Determining resources and financial support needed

4. Determining the roles and responsibilities of participants

5. Determining the availability and set-up of rooms and need for props, equipment, and actors (as necessary)

6. Preparing any handouts and materials required for the simulation exercise

The basic steps for conducting a simulation include:

1. Setting-up rooms/site for simulation including props, equipment, and other items required

2. Reviewing goals, desired outcomes of simulation, and a description of the scenario with participants

3. Reviewing of roles and responsibilities of participants

4. Conducting the actual simulation with participants

5. Conducting a debriefing with participants and reviewing lessons learned

An example of a scenario and outline for conducting a simulation of fire in the Operating Room is provided on the next page as a template.

EXAMPLE SCENARIO AND OUTLINE

DESCRIPTION	FIRE IN THE OR
GOAL/OUTCOMES	1. Review protocols for handling fire in the OR (RACE) 2. Prepare OR team to properly respond and handle fire in OR
PARTICIPANTS	▪ Surgeons ▪ Anesthesiologists ▪ Scrub techs ▪ Circulating Nurses ▪ Observer and note taker
SCENARIO	Patient is scheduled for surgery above the chest. Site is properly marked and patient is rated as high fire risk due to use of alcohol based prep and oxygen. Fumes pool under the drapes after patient prep and start a fire once the surgeon tries to use the cautery to stem some bleeding.
SUPPLIES NEEDED	▪ Dry ice to mimic smoke ▪ Red crepe paper to mimic fire
PRE EXERCRISE BRIEFING	▪ Review fire triangle ▪ Review RACE protocol
EXPECTED RESPONSES DURING SIMULATION	▪ Oxygen/gases turned off by Anesthesia provider ▪ Cautery turned off by surgeon ▪ Fire patted out by staff (if small), smothered with blanket or towel, and/or drapes removed from patient ▪ Ensure patient's immediate safety ▪ Ensure required care/treatment given to patient by team
DEBRIEFING	▪ Review what went well ▪ Review what didn't go well ▪ Review any changes needed

APPENDIX XIV

Customer Service Models

Quality of service often serves as a patient's proxy for the quality of care they receive from an organization or provider.

The use of service as a proxy for quality of care results from most patients lacking the medical knowledge and training needed to evaluate the appropriateness of clinical decisions.

Providing patients with extraordinary service is therefore critical for organizations and providers that want to be perceived as providing outstanding quality of care.

A number of different models are available for reinforcing with staff and providers the values and behaviors that help promote the delivery of outstanding service.

These models include FISH[202], AIDET[203] and the Caring model[204]

Another model is called I-CARE[SM] and is the acronym for:

I	**INTRODUCE**
C	**CAREFULLY LISTEN**
A	**ASK, ALTERNATIVES, ACT**
R	**REVIEW**
E	**ELICIT FEEDBACK** then **END**

202. Lundin, S. & Christensen, J. (2000). FISH! A Remarkable Way to Boost Morale and Improve Results. *Hyperion* March 2000

203. Studer, Q. (2003). Hardwiring Excellence. Studer Group 2003

204. The Caring Model, Caring Through Being
http://www.thecaringmodel.com/

A more detailed explanation of the I-CARE[SM, 205] service model along with examples is provided below:

I   **INTRODUCE** yourself and your role (as necessary) after extending a warm greeting to the patient

> *Clerical Example: Hi my name is Sue and I am the member services representative. How may I help you today?*

> *Clinical Example: Hi my name is John and I am the RN who will be taking care of you today. Do you have any pain or any concerns you would like me to help you with?*

C   **CAREFULLY LISTEN** to why the patient is there and **CONFIRM** what the patient is requesting or needs

> *Clerical Example: I understand you have been unable to schedule an appointment with a doctor and need help getting medical care.*

> *Clinical Example: I understand that the only immediate concern you have is the level of pain you are experiencing and need some pain medicine. Is that correct?*

A   **ASK** for additional information (if needed)

> *Clerical Example: Which doctor have you been trying to schedule your appointment with?*

> *Clinical Example: I see that they gave you ibuprofen last time you needed pain medicine. Did the ibuprofen help relieve your pain?*

    ADVISE of **ALTERNATIVES** (if needed)

> *Clerical Example: I will call Dr. Steven's module. If I am unable to schedule you with Dr. Stevens would you be willing for me to book you with another physician?*

205. I-CARE [SM] Service Model developed by Scott Lisbin

Clinical Example: If the ibuprofen did not sufficiently reduce your pain would you like me to contact the doctor to see if he will prescribe a stronger medicine?

ACT on agreed course of action

Clerical Example: I will call Dr. Steven's module now and see if he or another doctor can see you today.

Clinical Example: Since you said the ibuprofen worked last time to reduce your level of pain, I will go to the medicine room right now and return with a dose of valium to give you.

R   **REVIEW** what you have done to take care of the patient's needs or concerns

Clerical Example: I called Dr. Steven's module and he will be able to see you tomorrow.

Clinical Example: I have gotten a dose of ibuprofen that I will give to you now to help relieve your pain. You should start to feel some relief in about 30 minutes.

E   **ELICIT FEEDBACK** from the patient about their satisfaction with the action taken and anything else you can assist them with

Clerical Example: Will that be acceptable to you? Is there anything else I can assist you with?

Clinical Example: Please let me know if you still are experiencing pain after about half an hour. If so, I will see what else I can do to help relieve your pain. Is there anything else I can assist you with?

END with a departing remark

Example: I hope you feel better, or I hope you have a great rest of the day, etc.)

APPENDIX XV

TYPES OF CONTROL CHARTS

Different types of control charts are used to ensure statistical accuracy and appropriate decision-making when tracking data.

Control charts can be divided into two general categories depending on the type of data being collected and the size of the sample being taken; continuous (aka variable) control charts and attribute control charts.

Continuous control charts are used for tracking data that can be measured on a continuous scale (i.e., temperature, weight, etc.) while attribute control charts track data that are counted (i.e., items that are good or defective, pass or fail, or possess or do not possess a particular characteristic).

The "x-bar", "range R", and "S" control charts are used for tracking data that is considered continuous data.

The "x-bar" chart graphs the means or averages of a set of samples taken over time and demonstrates if the mean output of the process is changing over time.

The "range R" chart is used for relatively small sample sizes and tracks the variability within a process by measuring the difference between the smallest and largest readings.

The "S" chart is used for tracking the variation within a process when larger samples are required and measures the standard deviation between samples.

The "u" or "c" control charts are typically used when tracking "count" data such as the number of defects in a batch of raw materials or the number of defects in a finished product.

The "c" chart is typically used where there can be a number of defects per unit sampled and the number of units sampled per period remain constant.

The "u" chart is typically used when there can be a number of defects per unit sampled but the number of samples taken during the sampling period varies.

The "p" and "np" control charts are typically used when just a pass/fail determination is being made on a unit that is inspected.

The "p" chart is used when the sample size taken varies from observation to observation while the "np" chart is used when the sample size taken remains constant from observation/period to observation/period.

The following decision tree can be used to determine which type of control is most appropriate to use for the data being tracked.

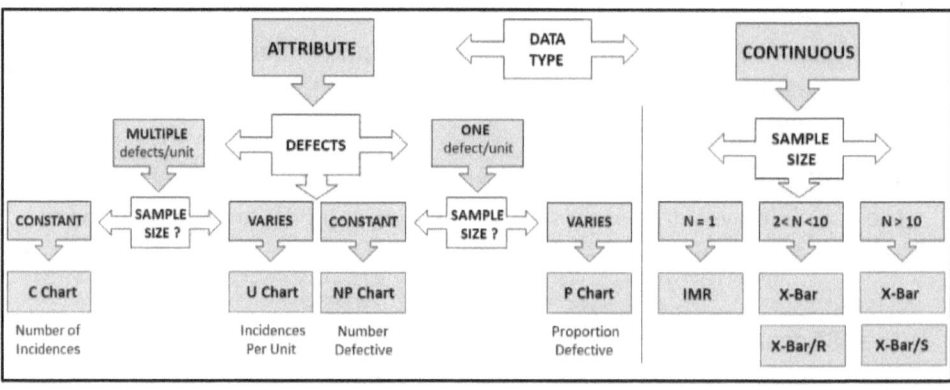

INDEX

5S   44, 176, 179-185
                        189, 198-200, 270
5 WHYs   52-55
Andon   74-76
Briefing   85-87, 235, 278
Channeling   73, 97-98
Checklists   72, 81, 87-88, 217-218
Cycle time   26, 77, 112, 118,
                        163-166, 170, 272-274
Defects   see waste
Drills   222, 277
Dynamic modeling   13, 18, 45-48
Fishbone diagram   52, 55-58
Feedback   13, 18, 37-40
Flowchart   20-27, 91, 92, 196, 256
FMEA   221-224
Gemba   13, 17-19
Goal alignment   202, 205-206
Handoffs   23, 63, 72, 80-87, 160,
                        170
Human talent   see waste
Inventory   see waste
Jidoka   72, 74-76
Just in time   139, 147-152, 202, 206-
                        207
Kanban   139, 153-156
Kubler Ross   239
Load level   100, 100-104, 157, 171-173
Motion   see waste
MUDA   1-3, 11, 13, 17-18, 20
                        24-25, 29-33, 35, 37, 41, 43
                        45-46, 51-55, 57-58, 60, 62
                        68, 71-72, 89, 99, 138, 163,
                        250
MURA   101, 103, 136, 166
MURI   104, 105, 108, 111, 163, 166
Nomogram   259, 261-262
One piece flow   133-137, 268-270
Overprocessing   see waste
Overproduction   see waste
Org culture   232-234
Pareto diagram   52, 58-62
PDCA/PDSA   12, 255
Poka-Yoke   72-74, 222, 224-226

Process map   13, 17-28
Production control   202-204
Preventive   222, 226-228
maintenance
Read back   81, 83-84
Repeat back   81, 83-84
Rounding   134, 245-246
Sample Size   43, 257, 259-262, 273, 283-
                        284
SBAR   82-84, 235
Sense of urgency   232, 234-238, 265
Service models   280-282
Simulations   13, 18, 45-48, 217, 222, 228-
                        230, 277-279
Six Sigma   13, 89, 231, 255
Small lot process   133, 136-137
SMED   120-124, 267
Standardized Work   72, 76-80, 270
TAKT time   25, 26, 77, 157, 163-170,
                        269, 274,
Transportation   see waste
Value Stream   13, 17, 25-30
Variation   33-36, 72, 89-90, 108, 139-
                        142, 165, 202-204, 255, 269,
                        271
Waiting   see waste
Waste
-Defects   3, 4, 27, 30, 53, 57, 61-63,
                        72-98, 157, 170, 171, 283,
                        284
-Human Talent   10, 11, 67, 68, 156-175,
-Inventory   7-9, 66, 67, 138-156, 195,
                        271
-Motion   7, 44, 65, 73, 74, 175-188
-Overprocessing   5, 6, 65, 209-217
-Overproduction   5, 64, 67, 202-209
-Transportation   8, 21, 64, 65, 151, 188-201
-Waiting   4, 5, 18, 19, 27, 46, 63, 99-
                        138, 144, 160, 207, 216, 263-
                        264, 273
Walk the Gemba   13, 17-19
Work Sampling   18, 29, 40-45, 259-262